HEALTHY LIFESTYLE FOR GOOD EYESIGHT

THE ULTIMATE GUIDE TO EYE CARE

Published July 2020

By

DR. MENMA A. OKECHUKWU

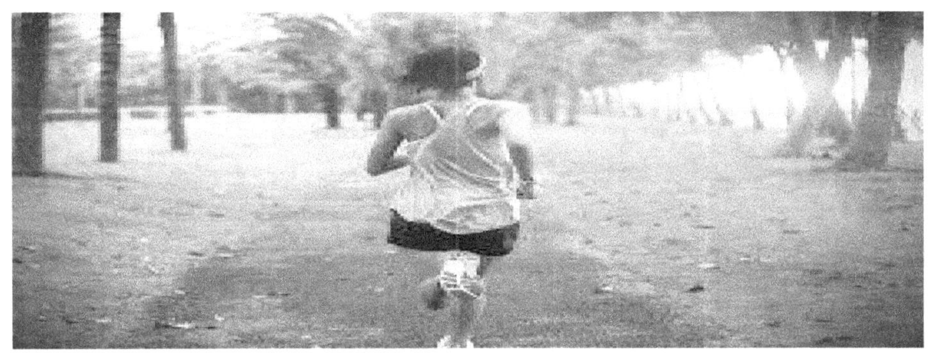

HEALTHY LIFESTYLE FOR GOOD EYESIGHT

THE ULTIMATE GUIDE TO EYE CARE

This book was written due to my passionate desire to create awareness about eye care, to let people know more about their eyes, and how to keep it safe. My goal is to create an informative book that is easy to read, for everyone. Pictures were used in this book to illustrate better for more understanding.

While all attempts have been made to verify the accuracy of the information provided in this book, the author assumes no responsibility for any error, omissions, or problems arising in connection with the health care guide provided in this book. For advice about your eyes and its health, please contact your eye care provider, if unavailable you can contact us via;
emmanuelcatholiceyeclinic@yahoo.com or
www.emmanuelcatholiceyeclinic.com/facebook.com

DR. MENMA A. OKECHUKWU

DEDICATED

To the Almighty God, my most faithful and adorable FATHER, who never gives up on me, for his infinite love, favors, and blessings. For His divine directions, I will forever worship you.

To my dearest parent, Sir Donatus and Lady Angelina Obiaghanwa who taught me that diligent, hard work and perseverance is the key to success and also for their unconditional love and efforts to make my life a success. I will be eternally grateful.

To my husband, Engr Stanley Okechukwu Udeobi for his love, support, and encouragement. Your enthusiastic spirit has made me achieve my dreams and has given me the desire to dream more. You are my very best from God. Thank you.

To my loving children, my bundles of joy, my treasures, for their patience and understanding.

CONTENT

CHAPTER 1: INTRODUCTION

The eye is one of the five sense organs, is an organ for sight. It's the most valuable sense organ, as 80% of what we perceive is from sight. Vision affects our quality of life greatly, is an essential part of everyday life for "sight is life, sight is wealth''.

Many body diseases cause changes in the eyes by their effect in vision, thus the eye is known as the window of the body, a healthy living is an important part of good vision.

Negligence of our eyesight may lead to loss of vision, we should, therefore, try to maintain and protect our precious sight, to enjoy many more years of good vision.

Kate: Good morning Doc,

Doctor: Good morning Kate, how are you today?

Kate: Doc am not happy with my eyes.

Doctor: What is the complain about?

Kate: Am just not comfortable with my vision. Doc, please are there foods or things I can do to keep my eyes healthy always?

Caring for your vision does not begin and end with glasses, contact lens and eye surgeries, your health is wrapped up in your lifestyle and gene so overall care is essential.

As it's important to keep your body healthy, you also need to keep your eyes healthy, for "a healthy eye is a healthy body''.

CHAPTER 2: ANATOMY OF THE EYES

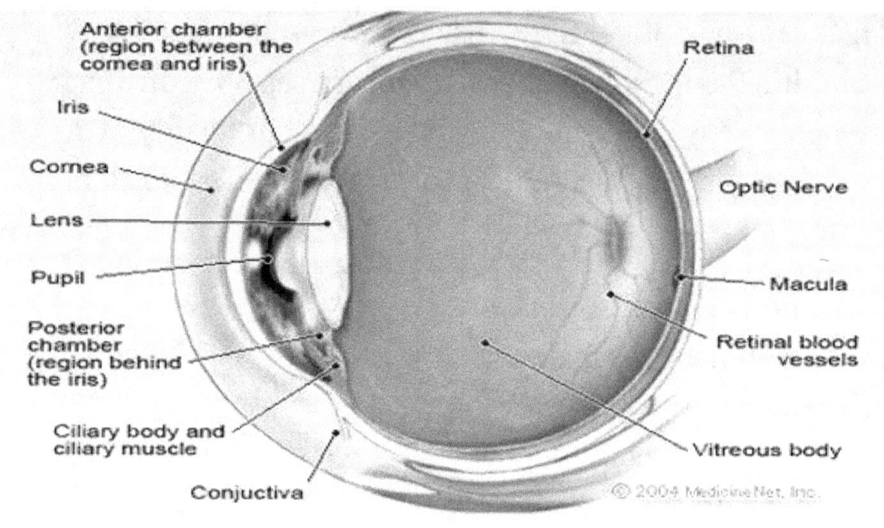

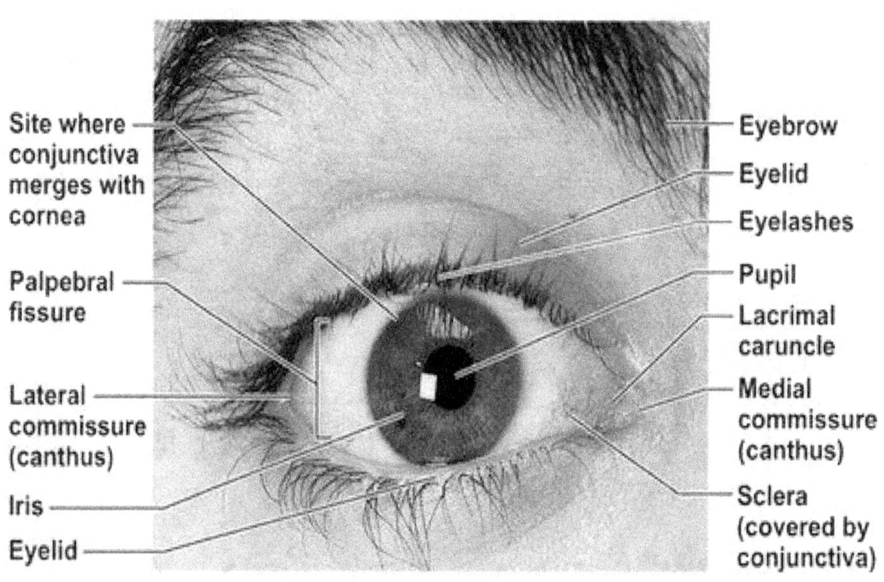

The anatomy of the eye is complex. The main structures of the eye include;

- Cornea: clear tissue in the very front of the eye.

- Iris: colored part of the eye surrounding the pupil.

- Pupil: a dark hole in the iris that regulates the amount of light going into the eye.

- Lens: small clear disk inside the eye that focuses light rays onto the retina.

- Retina: the layer that lines the back of the eye, senses light, and creates electrical impulses that travel through the optic nerve to the brain.

- Macula: small central area in the retina that allows us to see fine details.

- Optic nerve: connects the eye to the brain and carries the electrical impulses formed by the retina to the visual cortex of the brain.

- Vitreous: a clear, jelly-like substance that fills the middle of the eye.

CHAPTER 3: HYGIENE

3.1. HAND HYGIENE

Our hands harbor germs and bacteria that can cause eye infections, thus proper cleansing is essential to ensure eye health.

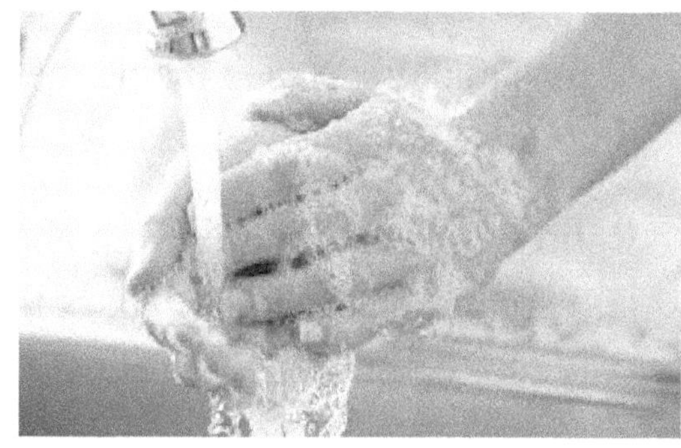

Avoid common eye infections by proper washing of the hands before touching your face or eyes.

We tend to rub our eyes, when our eyes are irritated like itching, feeling of foreign body sensation, infection, or allergies.

Rubbing our eye might damage it especially the cornea, this could result in an infection and may transfer infection from the hand to the eyes.

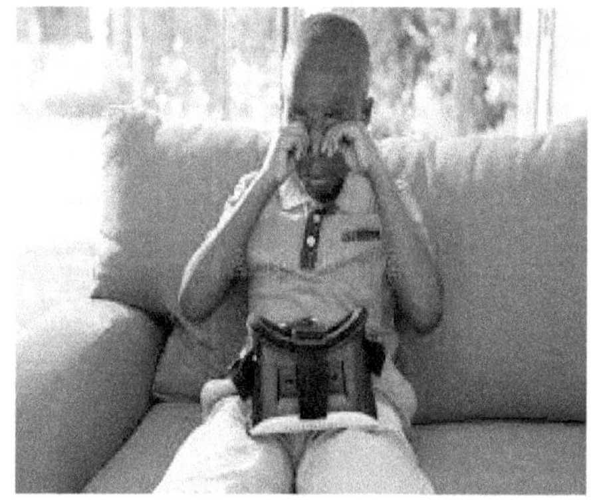

If you have allergies and your eyes itch, rubbing your eyes can release more histamine (allergens) into the areas around your eyes, thereby increasing itching.

Rubbing our eyes can cause tiny blood vessels to break, resulting in bloodshot eyes and dark unsightly circles under the eyes.

Flush the eyes with lukewarm water to remove dirt, sand, or loose eyelashes from your eyes. Place a cold compress over your eyes if the itchy, swollen, or red. However, the best way to stop rubbing your eyes is to treat the underlying cause by visiting your eye doctor.

Make regular washing of hands a habit, like washing your hands; after shaking hands with someone, before and after eating, after using the toilet, after any activity or work to avoid infections.

Guide for proper handwashing; wash your palm, wrist, back of your hands, under your fingernails and between the fingers with soap and clean water, then dry with a clean towel.

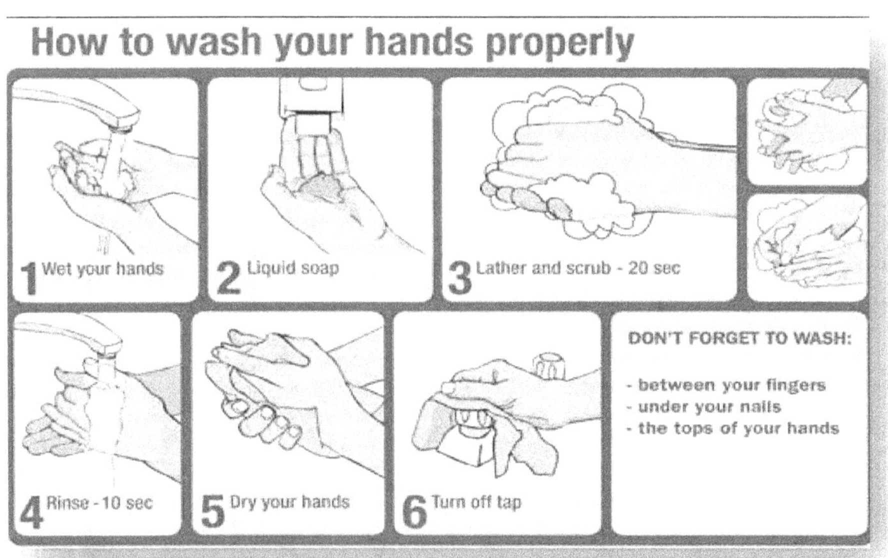

3.2. FACIAL HYGIENE

Bacteria, dirt, and other foreign particles on the face can sometimes get in contact with the eyes.

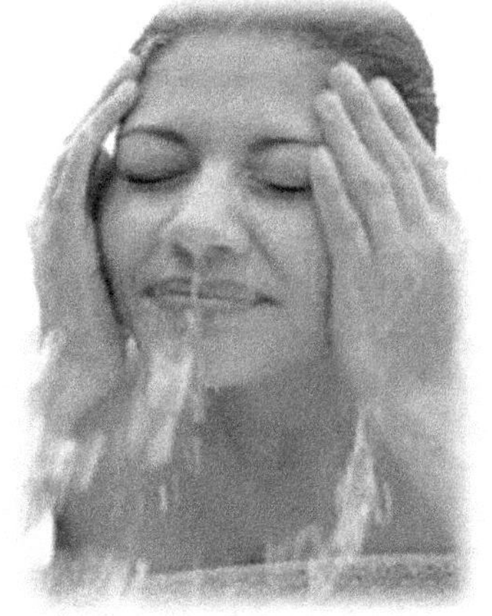

It's important to wash the face with clean water and soap to prevent the eyes from becoming infected due to its exposure to germs and bacteria and dry with a fresh clean towel.

Use a clean handkerchief or face towel to clean your face especially, when sweating, and avoid using the same face towel for coughing, sneezing, or cleaning the nose, to avoid infecting the eyes.

Avoid sharing towels and makeups to prevent getting your eyes vulnerable to contagious eye infections, since germs that cause eye diseases thrive in moist and dark environment.

Liquid and creamy eye makeup may harbor bacteria, discard makeup, and mascara every 3months.

Wash your face properly and clean off your makeups before sleeping, for excess debris from makeup can cause eye irritation and redness.

Always use quality eye makeup to prevent irritating the eyes.

To clean off your makeup, use warm compresses, makeup wipes, or natural good alternatives like coconut oil.

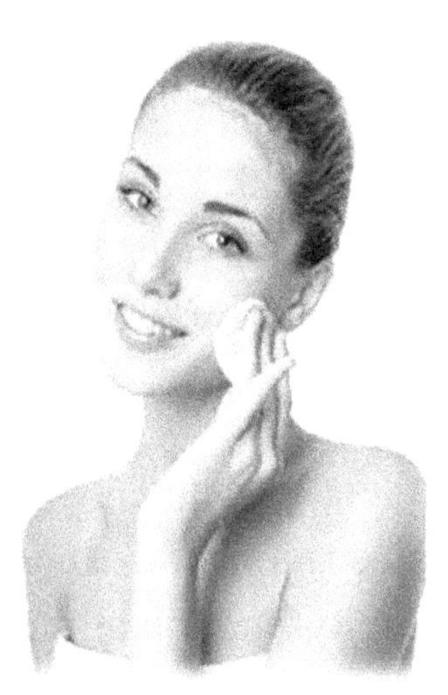

If your experiencing allergies or eye irritations do not use eye makeup because this could increase redness, itching, and make you rub your eyes.

If you get an eye infection, please discard your eye makeup and visit an eye doctor.

3.3. SLEEP HYGIENE

For physical and mental health quality and regular sleep is essential, for sleep is a vital indicator of overall health and wellbeing.

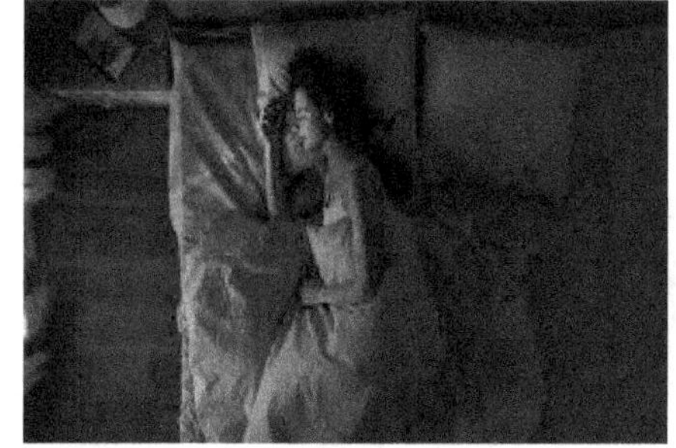

Adults needs about 7 to 9 hours of sleep and children require more, to function at their best, however, studies show that the eyes need at least 5 hours of sleep per night to properly replenish.

Adequate sleep ensures that your eyes are well-rested and strain-free. Skimping on sleep can affect how well your eyes work, it could become puffy, red, and tired.

If you do not get enough sleep, your eyes might not produce the tears necessary to clean and moisture themselves, leading to dry eyes.

You feel tired and strained when you go for a long period without sleep and your vision seems blurry and it almost hurts to keep your eyes open.

Lack of sleep causes dark circles or bags to form under your eyes; this is because a lack of sleep tends to increase the retention of blood and fluid around the eyes.

Sleep deprivation can cause eye spasms (involuntary eye twitching), which can be uncomfortable and distracting. Getting adequate rest can assist in eyesight improvement since sleep allows overworked eye muscles to relax completely.

An extended amount of sleep deprivation has been attributed to causing anterior ischemic optic neuropathy (an inflammatory disease of the blood vessels which can lead to vision loss) especially in middle age to elderly, who suffer from a history of sleep apnea.

TIPS FOR GETTING THE SLEEP YOU NEED

- Dim the light in your room about an hour before bed to signal your body and mind that it is time to sleep.
- Exercising regularly during the day can help you sleep much better, do not exercise within 3 hours of trying to get to sleep, for it can make sleeping difficult.
- Have a regular schedule for sleeping; it will help your body regulate your sleep and your energy levels.
- Sleep in a quiet, cool, and dark environment, try to avoid noisy areas and put off your screens, you may consider wearing a face mask.

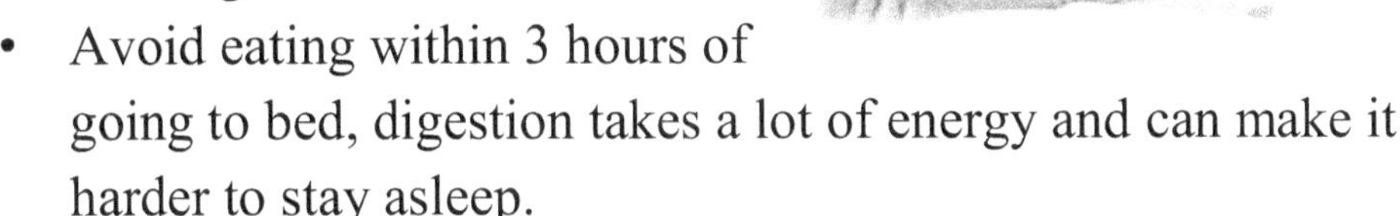

- Avoid eating within 3 hours of going to bed, digestion takes a lot of energy and can make it harder to stay asleep.

Avoid caffeine and alcohol before going to bed.

Visit your eye doctor, if you have problems sleeping.

3.4. DOMESTIC HYGIENE

Keep your home free from dust and avoid exposing your eyes to dust, dust irritates the eyes and may cause harm to the eyes.

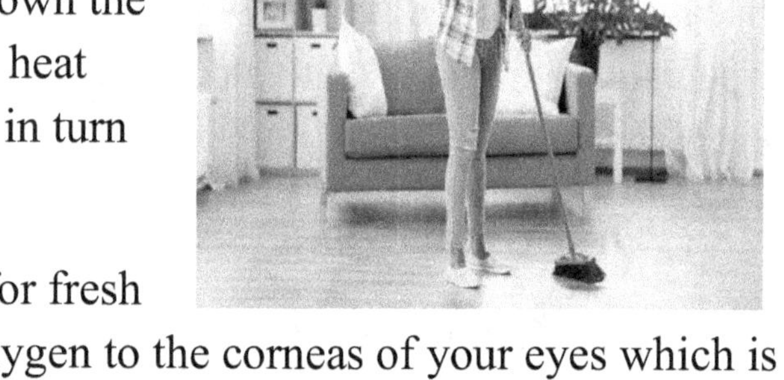

It's advisable to turn down the heat in your house, for heat dries out the air which in turn dries out your eyes.

Keep your home airy for fresh air directly supplies oxygen to the corneas of your eyes which is beneficial for its good health.

Our eyes need a certain level of moisture from the air around us to produce tears and prevent dryness, for serious dryness can lead to corneal abrasion and even blindness.

Avoid exposing your eyes to dry air like an air conditioner, it dries out the moisture out of your eyes, so it's good to turn the vents away from your face and use it with moderation.

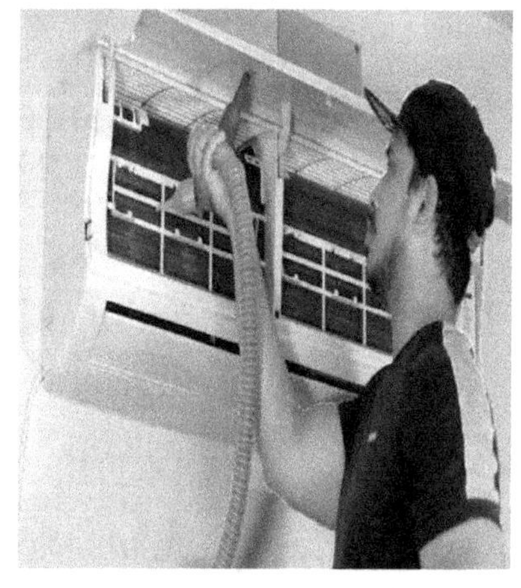

Air conditioners reduce humidity and cause evaporative dry eye, resulting in redness, itching, irritation, and eye strain. Clean your AC vents, for it harbors molds, bacteria, and viruses which can cause eye inflammation.

Pets like dogs, cats, or even birds can cause allergic eye reactions like itching, tearing, redness, puff eyelid.

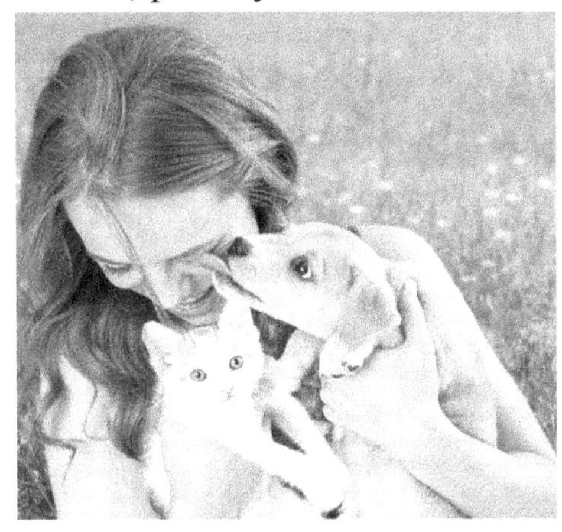

These allergies can be gotten from pet dander (dead skin cells), saliva, urine, pollen, thus it is advisable not to spend a lot of time around them or sleep with them, especially for those who are allergic.

Always wash your hands and clothes, after being in contact with pets, however, it's wise to take a bath.

Keep your home neat always, it's better to use a central air cleaner, if you have pets in the house to minimize blowing allergens throughout the house. Keep your pet's environment clean and place the litter box away from vents or choose a place not connected to your central air.

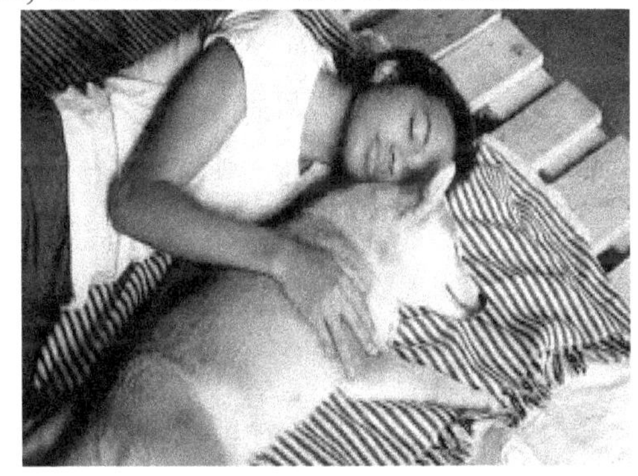

Most importantly, avoid touching your eyes and face after coming in contact with pets.

3.5. CONTACT LENS HYGIENE

A contact lens is a convenient and comfortable alternative to eyeglasses for many people.

Contact lens is safe for vision correction or cosmetics purposes when you follow the proper care and wearing instruction provided by your eye doctor to avoid eye infections especially blindness.

Contact lens is a thin, curved lens, made from different types of plastics, placed on the films of tears that cover the surface of your eyes.

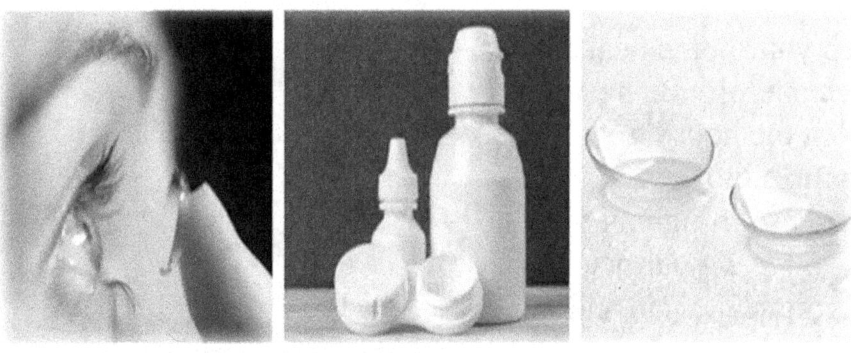

There are different types of contact lens never buy any without your doctor's permission and prescription, for different types, require knowledge about its special care, length of time to be worn, and certain types of product.

Contact lens provides many health benefits, but they are not risk-free, your eye doctor can help you understand how to get the full benefits of your contact lens and reduce your chances of developing eye problems.

People who wear contact lens have a higher risk of having corneal diseases with severe pain, which can cause vision loss, so it's essential to keep to the rules of contact lens.

Hygiene is the most critical aspect of successful long-term contact lens wear. Always wash and dry your hands before handling the contact lens and follow your doctor's guide for contact lens insertion and removal.

It's good to keep your fingernails short and smooth to avoid damaging your lenses or scratching the eye while inserting or removing contact lens.

Rub the contact lens with your fingers gently and rinse them thoroughly before soaking the lenses overnight in a multipurpose solution that completely covers each lens.

Store lenses in the proper lens storage case, clean the case after each use, and keep it to dry. Always use fresh solutions to clean and store contact lens.

Replace your contact lens case every 3 months or sooner, for studies show that storage cases are contaminated with invisible microbes, thus regular replacement is your best defense from getting your eyes infected.

Use the recommended contact lens wetting solution, do not use water, saliva, or expired solution, and never reuse old solutions.

Always follow the recommended contact lens replacement schedule prescribed by your doctor.

Do not sleep in contact lenses that are not approved for overnight wear, and do not use disposable contact lenses beyond their wear.

Do not wear other people's contact lenses to avoid the spread of infections and not shower or swim with contact lenses.

If you wear contact lenses you should be examined by an eye doctor annually or more often as needed.

Take your lenses off and visit your eye doctor if you experience, redness, pain, increased light sensitivity, itching, discharge, or your vision changes.

If you do not use lenses as directed, you could be damaging your eyes. Clean and safe handling of your contact lens is one of the most important things you can do to protect your sight.

CHAPTER 4: NUTRITION

4.1. FOOD

Healthy eyes provide good vision which is essential for an enjoyable and productive lifestyle.

A good diet plays a vital role in human health with no exception to the eyes.

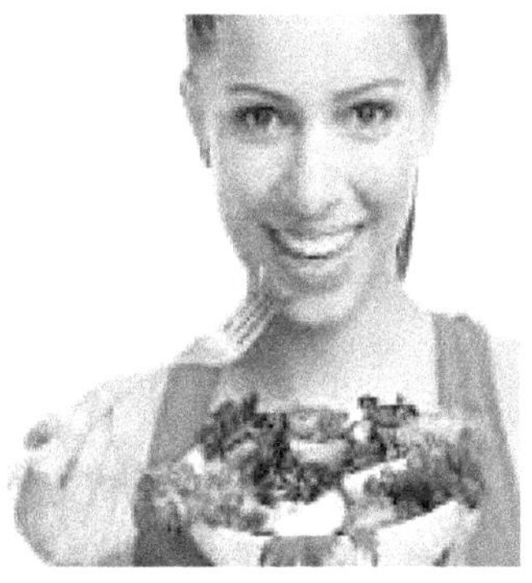

A balanced diet gives you a better chance of living healthy with healthy eyes.

Eating healthy foods will help you reduce your risk of developing eye diseases such as cataracts, (which causes cloudy vision) age-related macular degeneration (which affects your central vision), glaucoma, dry eyes, poor night vision.

A balanced diet is best created with a variety of proteins, dairy, fruits, and vegetables.

Limit consumption of unhealthy foods that are processed, contain saturated fats or are high in sugar.

Your eyes require antioxidants like **lutein, zeaxanthin, vitamin (A, C, E), beta-carotene, omega-3 fatty acid, zinc,** they all play different roles in promoting the health of your eyes.

Foods that contain these antioxidants include;

- LUTEIN

Egg, spinach, collard greens, kale, romaine lettuce, squash.

- ZEAXATHIN

Egg, spinach, collard greens, kale, romaine lettuce, squash, turnip greens, broccoli, peas.

- VITAMIN A

Dark green leafy vegetables such as turnip greens, spinach, broccoli, peas, red grapes, yellow squash, oranges, corn, mangoes, honeydew, lemon, liver, egg, milk, yogurt, carrot, bell pepper.

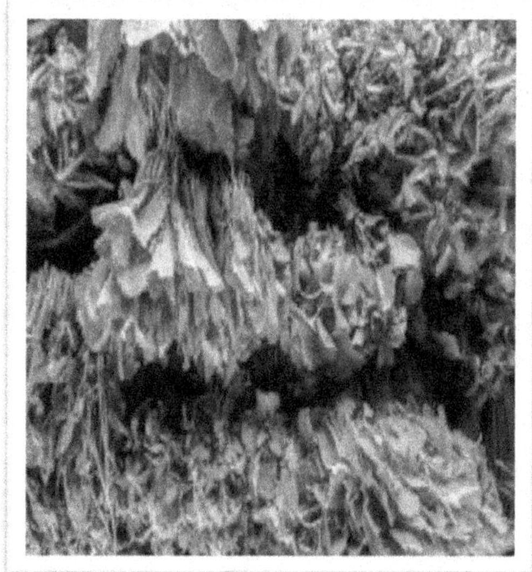

- VITAMIN C

Sweet potatoes, citrus (orange, grapefruits, tangerine, lemon), watermelon, berries, bell pepper, strawberries, broccoli, cantaloupe, kale, peaches, tomatoes, pawpaw.

- VITAMIN E

Walnuts, almonds, sunflower seeds, hazelnuts, peanuts, avocados, kale, spinach, collard green

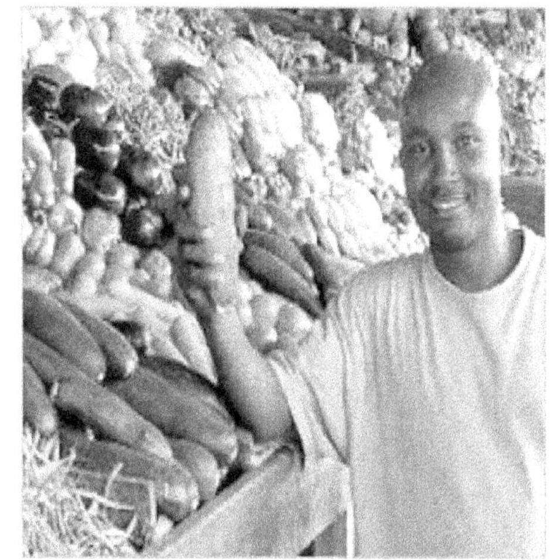

- BETACAROTENE

Kale, mangoes, cantaloupe, apricots, pawpaw, carrots, sweet potatoes, butternut, squash, dark green fruits including spinach and collard greens.

- OMEGA-3 FATTY ACIDS

Fish, (salmon, sardines, mackerel, tuna, herring), walnuts, almonds, chars' seeds, halibut, trout.

- ZINC

Legumes, (black-eyed peas, kidney beans, lima beans), milk, egg, yogurt, shellfish, like oysters, beef, lean red meat, poultry, fortified cereals.

Garlic, onions, soy is also very good for the eyes, they help prevent the formation of cataracts and improve the lens health of your eyes, they also help reduce inflammation in and around the eyes.

Your eyes are unique and have their own set of nutritional needs, however, to meet this need, some eye antioxidants supplements are designed to provide a balanced combination of nutrients essential for healthy eyes.

4.2. WATER: HYDRATION

Water is needed for various organs to function well; the body becomes dehydrated when more water leaves the body than enters it.

Inadequate hydration causes our organs including the eyes to suffer.

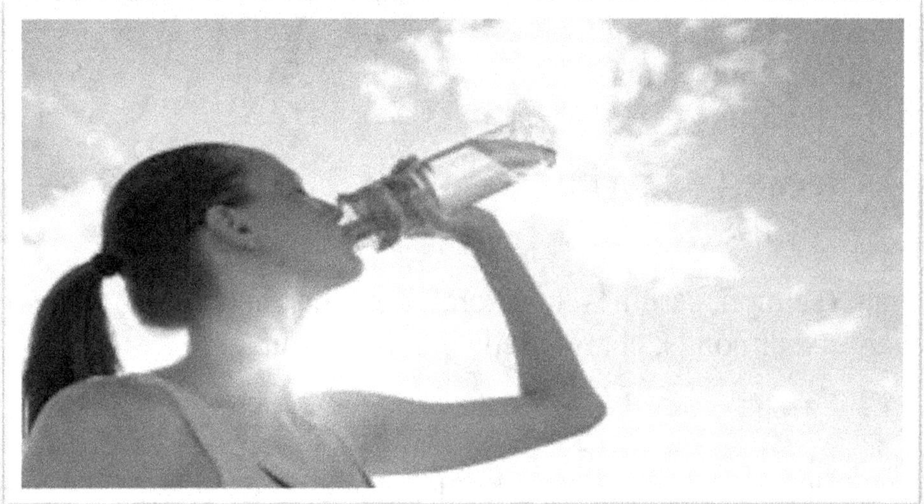

Fluid loss occurs in daily bodily functions, such as heat, urination, and bowel movements, also extreme heat, vomiting, diarrhea, alcohol, and even diabetes increases the risk of dehydration.

When the body is dehydrated, its essential response is to preserve the amount of fluid still in the body, and for the eyes, it leads to a lack of tear production.

Lack of tear production causes the eyes not to be well lubricated, which can lead to dry eyes, eye strain, and other vision problems.

Tears are necessary to provide clear vision, wash away foreign matters in the eyes, and help reduce the risk of eye infection.

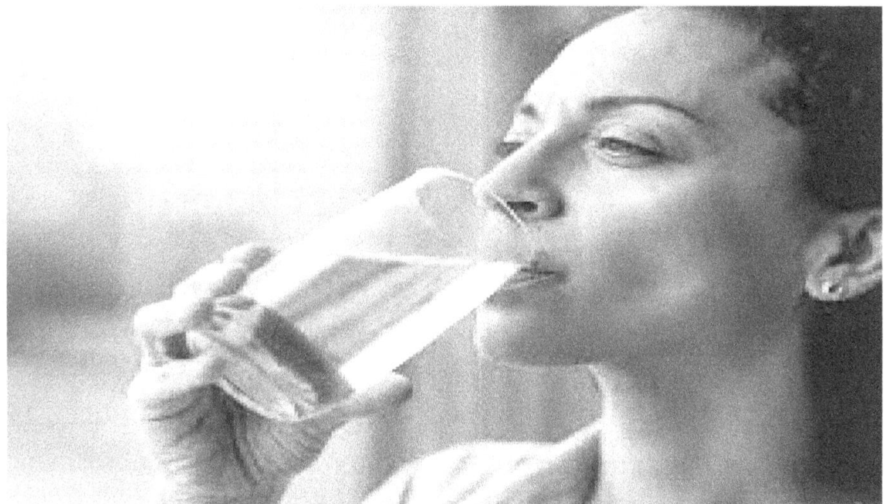

Maintaining health eyes by drinking water can also prevent eye floaters and flush out the toxins, that form them, thus getting rid of them.

Drinking a lot of water (about 2.5 liters), throughout the day, can prevent dehydration.

Dehydration can also be prevented by reducing your salt intake, alcohol, caffeine, and high protein foods intake, also your stress level.

4.3. CAFFEINE INTAKE

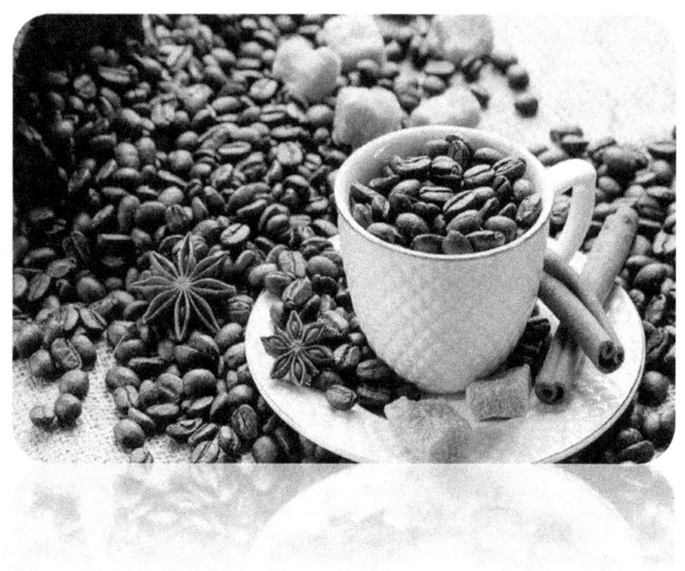

Caffeine is a natural stimulant most commonly found in tea, coffee, cocoa plants, soft drinks, and energy drinks.

It stimulates the brain and central nervous system and helps you to stay alert and prevent the onset of tiredness.

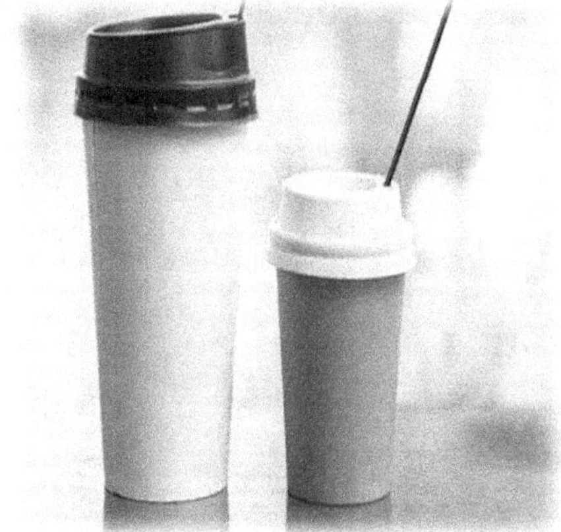

Too much caffeine may promote headaches, migraines, high blood pressure in some individuals.

Excessive caffeine can negatively impact your vision in the short term, and over time can cause more serious damage.

Excessive consumption of caffeine affects our vision, it can suddenly increase sugar levels, which can lead to blurred vision or spasms of the eyelid.

Reduction in tear production has also been linked with consuming large amounts of caffeine in a short period, causing dry eyes, symptoms being, eye discomfort, burning, or gritty sensation.

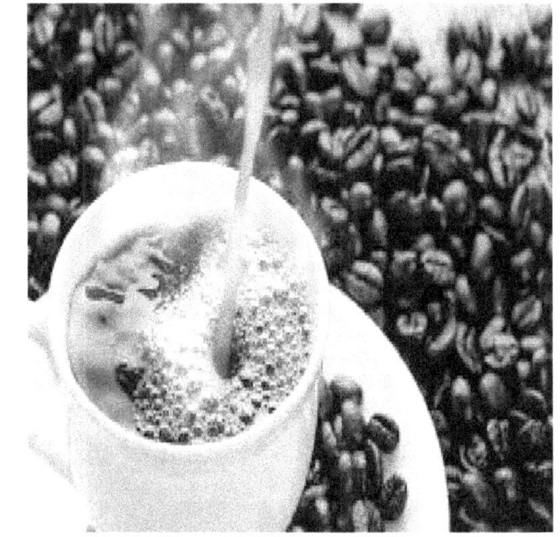

According to research, regular consumption of 3 or more cups of coffee per day would contribute to the accumulation of deposits inside the eyes called "exfoliation", which may put you at risk of getting glaucoma.

Caffeine consumption is generally considered safe when taken in moderation.

4.4. GREEN TEA INTAKE

Green tea is one of the healthiest beverages, is a type of tea that is made from Camellia Sinensis leaves and buds that have not undergone the same withering and oxidation process used to make oolong teas and black teas.

It contains a catechin called epigallon-catechin-3-gallate(EGCG), polyphenols, less caffeine.

Catechins are antioxidants, that protect the eyes, they are absorbed by different parts of the eye like the retina, lens, and other eye tissues.

Green tea is loaded with antioxidants that are beneficial to the body. It helps in the eye, heart, and brain function, it protects against cancer, fat loss, lowers high cholesterol levels.

Green tea is packed with powerful eye-healthy nutrients like catechin, which can improve eyesight and prevent eye diseases like cataracts, macular degeneration, glaucoma, dry eyes.

It protects the retina, lens, and aqueous humor, it also protects the eyes from ultraviolet rays (sun) and harmful blue light.

Green tea consumption could benefit the eyes against oxidative stress and inflammation.

Limit your green tea consumption to 2-3 cups per day, because in excess it can lead to undesirable effects.

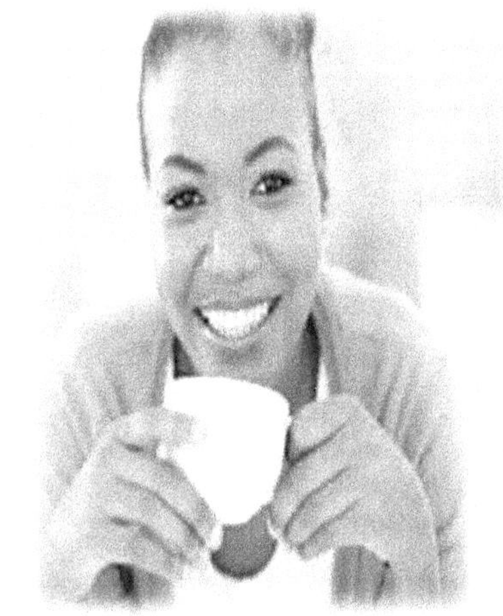

Green tea is not recommended for some individuals like pregnant and breastfeeding moms and those with high blood pressure, insomnia.

4.5. ALCOHOLIC DRINKING

Alcoholic drink is a drink that contains the drug ethanol, which is produced by fermentation of grains, fruits, or other sources of sugar.

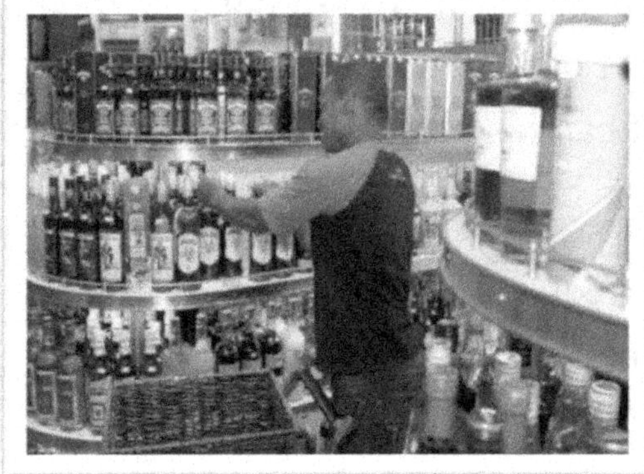

Alcohol can be found in drinks like beer, wine, and spirits(liquor) and it can be toxic and addictive.

It is a depressant, meaning it slows down the messages that travel between your brain and your body and affects the way you think, feel, and behave.

Prolonged and excessive intake of alcohol affects your body and vision.

Alcohol slower pupil reaction, it causes the iris to constrict and dilate at a much slower speed, making light-dark adaptation (changing from a bright environment to a dark environment) difficult.

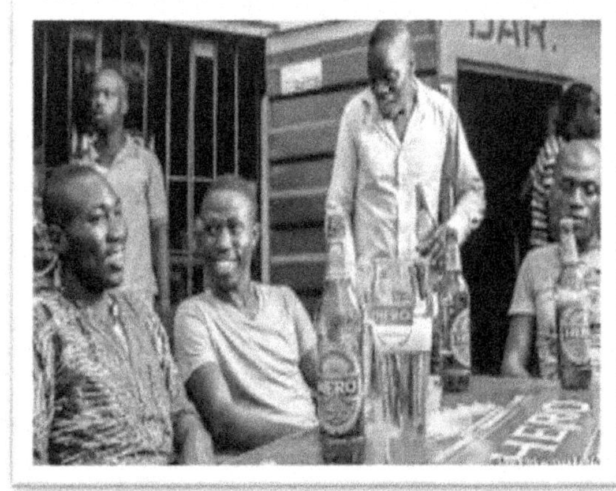

It decreases contrast sensitivity, which is impairing the ability to distinguish between different objects based on light and darkness.

It causes eyelid twitching, increased eye dryness, bloodshot and sore eyes, double vision, blurry vision, extreme sensitivity to light, and can cause migraine headaches.

Alcohol intake can increase cataract formation, increase the risk of age-related macular degeneration.

It decreases vision due to vitamin deficiency because heavy drinking affects the absorption of vitamins in the liver, which are needed to maintain healthy eyesight. Vitamin deficiency will lead to weakness or paralysis of the eye muscles, night blindness, thinning of the cornea, corneal perforation, severe dryness, and even blindness due to retinal damage.

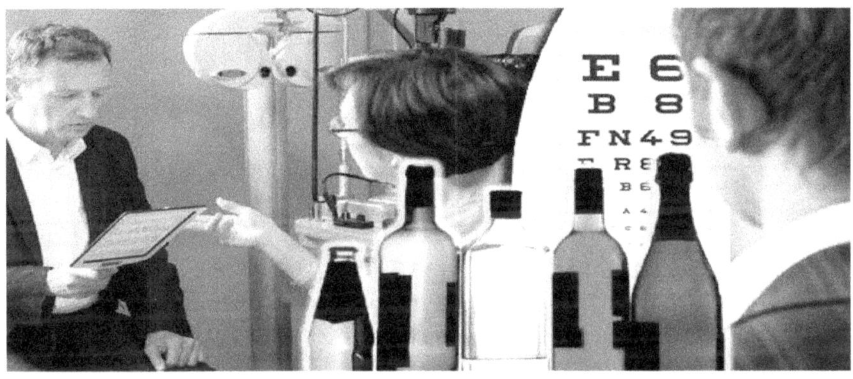

Studies have also shown an increased risk of developing various forms of neuropathy or nerve damage, including optic neuropathy, this condition can cause loss of vision, decrease in peripheral vision, and color vision.

Excessive exposure to alcohol in the womb can permanently affect the eyesight of the baby causing fetal alcohol syndrome, which includes underdevelopment of the optic nerve, difficulty with eye coordination, and the tendency for the eyelid to drop.

For pregnant or breastfeeding mothers not drinking is the safest option.

There may be potential beneficial effects of alcohol drinking, however, for a better and healthy sight, light to moderate amount of alcohol is advised. Moderate drinking means up to 1 drink a day for women and 2 drinks a day for men.

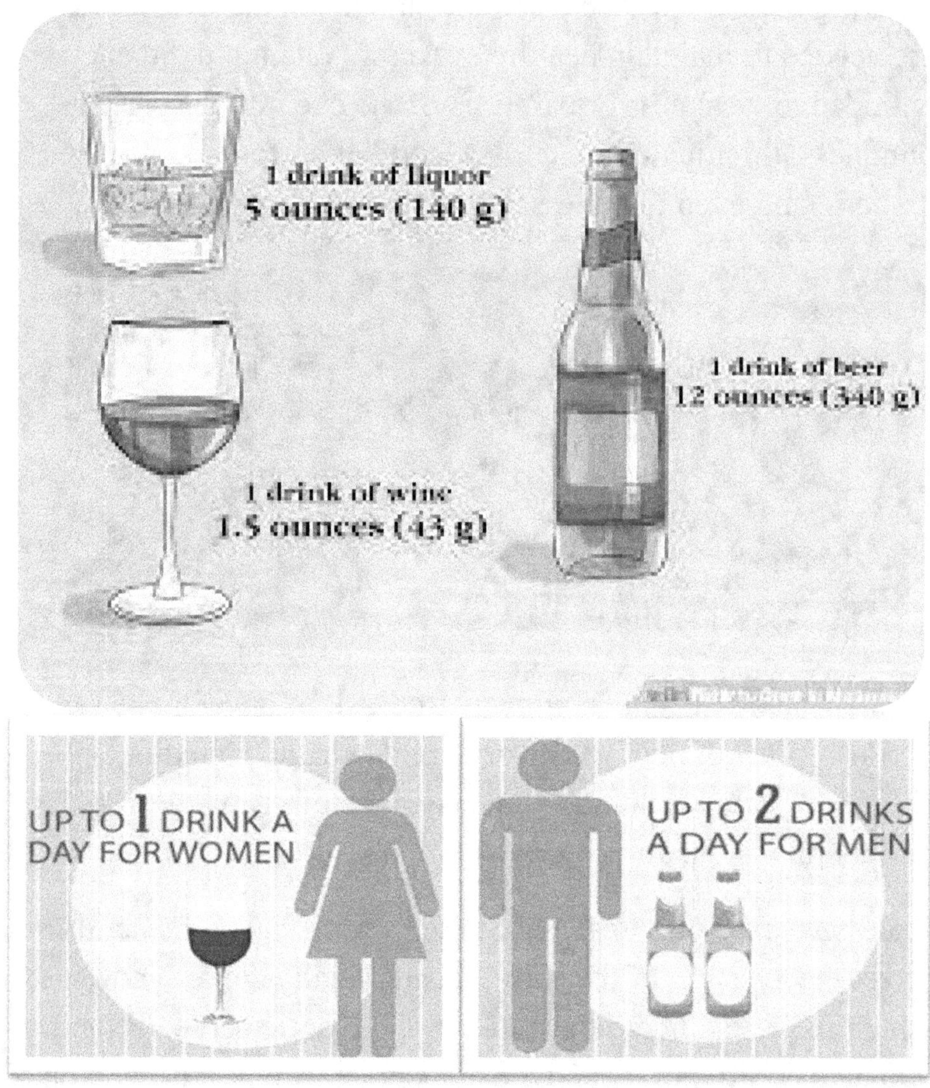

4.6. SMOKING

Smoking is the act of inhaling and exhaling the fumes of burning plant materials like tobacco as smoked in a cigarette, cigar or pipe, marijuana, and hashish, into the bloodstream.

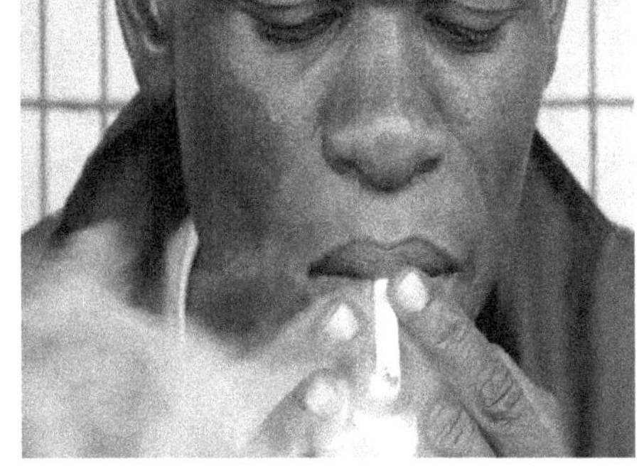

Tobacco smoking is the most popular, it's dangerous to our health, toxic, highly addictive, and a stimulant.

Components of tobacco smoke include nicotine, carbon monoxide, reactive oxygen species, heavy metals examples cadmium, and lead.

Smoking is the single largest preventable cause of diseases and death, it harms nearly every organ in your body including your eyes.

Smoking causes negative biological changes in your eyes, thus avoiding smoking or taking steps to quit, lowers your risk of vision impairment or vision loss.

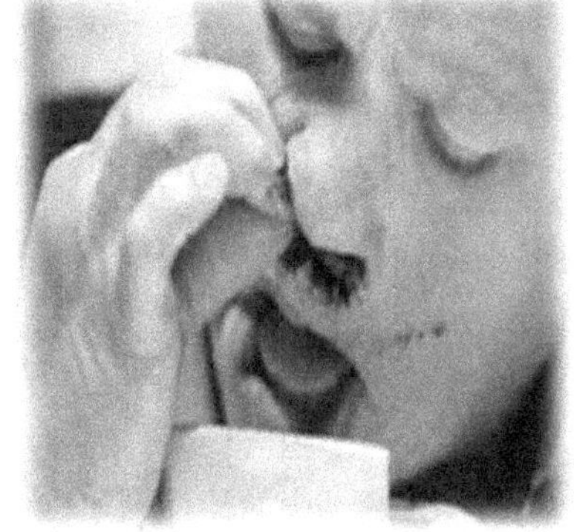

Tobacco can be chewed, sucked, dissolved, or inhaled through the mouth or nose, using other forms of tobacco often known as chewing tobacco, oral tobacco, snuff, or sinus.

Chemicals present in tobacco can damage the eye's blood vessels and lead to an acute constriction of the ciliary arteries, which reduces the blood flow to eyes.

Nicotine and carbon monoxide accelerates atherosclerosis and interferes with lipid homeostasis causing fatty deposits in the blood vessels. Noxious particles present in tobacco smoking acts as irritants to the conjunctiva.

Smoking affects your health, even if you don't breathe in the smoke, and also affects the people around you through your second-hand smoke.

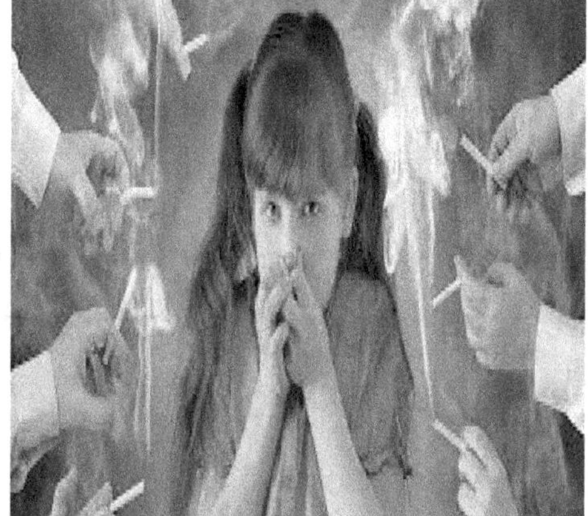

Smoking causes tear film instability and lead to a decrease in tear break up time, decreased corneal and conjunctival sensitivity.

It increases platelet aggregations and can induce blood clotting, if these processes affect the ophthalmic branch of the carotid vasculature, this can cause ocular ischemic episodes.

Tobacco smoke contains free radicals that reduce the presence of protective antioxidants leading to oxidative damage to the retina.

Heavy metals such as cadmium, lead, copper found in tobacco smoke can accumulate in the lens of the eyes causing cataract formation.

Smokers are at higher risk of developing; age macular degeneration, cataract, uveitis, thyroid eye disease, dry eyes, optic neuropathy, diabetic retinopathy, abnormal eye movements (nystagmus, strabismus), and amblyopia.

Smoking should be strictly avoided by pregnant mothers, for the dangerous effects of smoking are transmitted through the placenta and the health and development of the offspring are affected.

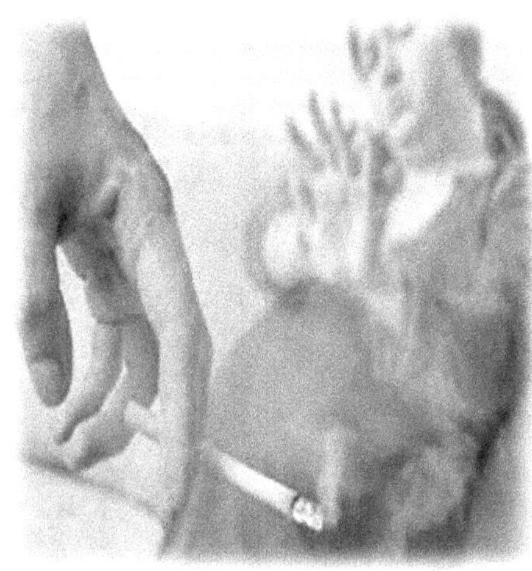

Quitting smoking or not starting in the first place and eliminating exposure to environmental tobacco smoking are the key ways to ensure that good vision is maintained for as long as possible.

It is not easy to quit smoking, but it is worth it, for the sake of your eyes and overall health.

CHAPTER 5: MEDICAL CARE

5.1. COMPREHENSIVE EYE EXAM

Your eyes need specialized care because they are one of the most sophisticated organs in your body.

You might think that your vision is fine or that your eyes are healthy but visiting your eye care professional for a comprehensive and dilated eye exam is the only way to be sure.

Many common eye diseases such as glaucoma, diabetic eye diseases, and age-related macular degeneration often have no warning signs, a dilated eye exam is the only way to detect these diseases in their early stages, left untreated they can cause serious vision loss and blindness.

Comprehensive eye exams not only test your vision but also gives the eye doctor a close up look at the inside of the eye, including blood vessels and nerves, all of which may contain clues to conditions that affect your overall health.

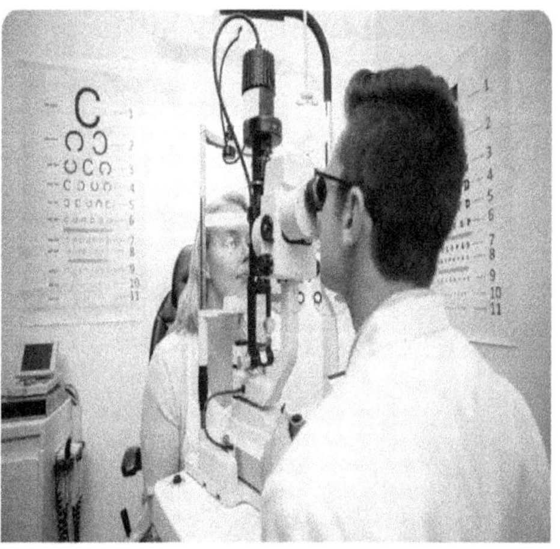

When it comes to vision problems, some people don't know they could see better with glasses or contact lenses.

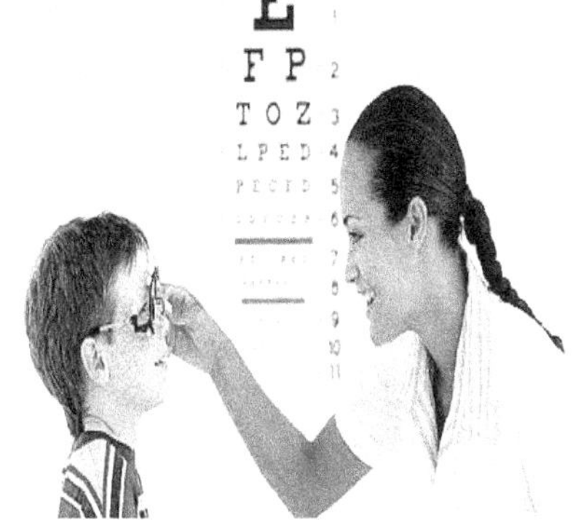

Be vigilant about your eyesight and keep looking for any changes in your vision.

Some of the signs and symptoms include; cloudy vision, blurry vision, double vision, redness, itching, discharges, tearing, floaters, flashes of light, eye ache, pain, headache, etc. If any of these signs and symptoms prevail consult your eye doctor.

Eyes are sensitive indicators and show up health problems long before there are any obvious physical symptoms.

Most eye diseases can be quite serious, which means that a comprehensive eye exam can help save your sight, early intervention now will prevent vision loss later.

Comprehensive eye exam might include;

- Visual acuity test; you read an eye chart about 20feet away, to check how well you see at various distances.

- Refraction (glasses test); to determine long-sightedness, short-sightedness, astigmatism, and presbyopia.

- External eye exam; which involves an examination of the anterior part of the eyes (eyelid, conjunctiva, cornea, anterior chamber, pupil) including the face.

- Microscopic eye examination before and after dilation (which involves putting dilating eye drops into the eye to widen the pupil, to aid a clearer view of important tissues at the back of the eye, including the retina, macular and optic nerve).

- Tonometry; to determine the intraocular pressure of your eyes. It helps to detect glaucoma.

- Visual field test; to measure your side (peripheral) vision. A loss of peripheral vision may be a sign of glaucoma.

- Finally, diagnosis, treatment, and /or management.

A comprehensive eye exam is recommended for at least every one to two years, depending on your age, risk factors, and whether you currently wear glasses or contacts.

However, you should get your eyes checked as often as your eye care provider recommends it, or if you have any vision problems. Ocular manifestation is often the presenting signs of life-threatening systemic diseases, thus comprehensive eye exam can save not only your sight but also your life.

5.2. EYE CARE PROVIDERS

Eye care providers are professionals trained to safeguard your precious sense of sight and help you maintain a lifetime of good vision. Ophthalmologist, optometrist, and opticians are the three main eye care professionals; however, each has different levels of training and expertise.

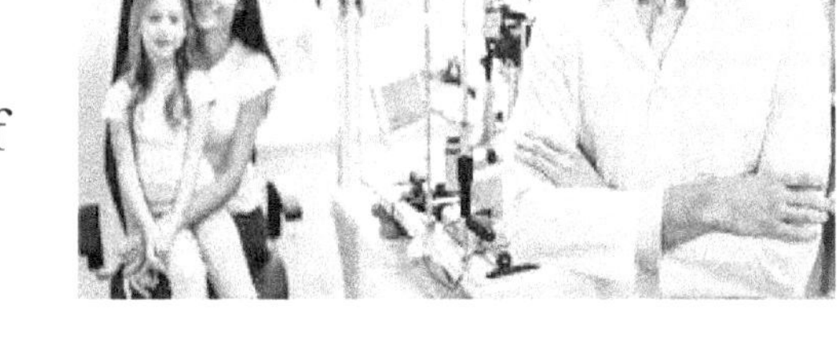

An ophthalmologist is a medical doctor, who specializes in the comprehensive care of the eyes and visual system in the prevention of eye diseases and injury. They examine, diagnose, and treat eye diseases, prescribe medications, and perform surgery. They also prescribe glasses and contact lens.

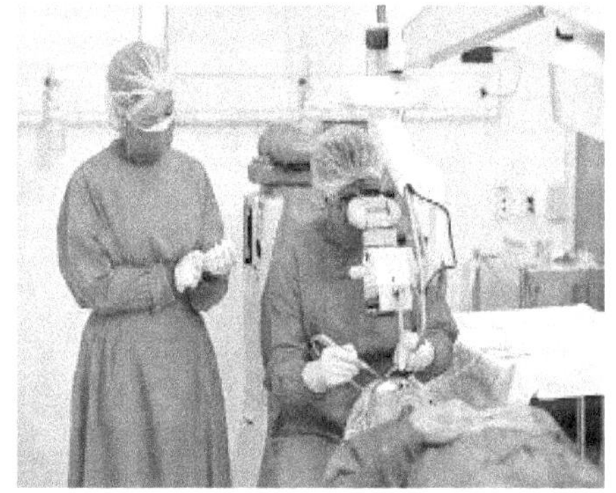

An optometrist is an eye doctor, who has earned the doctor of optometry degree. They specialize in comprehensive eye health, vision examinations, diagnosis, and treatment/management of eye diseases and vision disorders by prescribing medications, glasses, and contact lens. However, they do not perform surgeries.

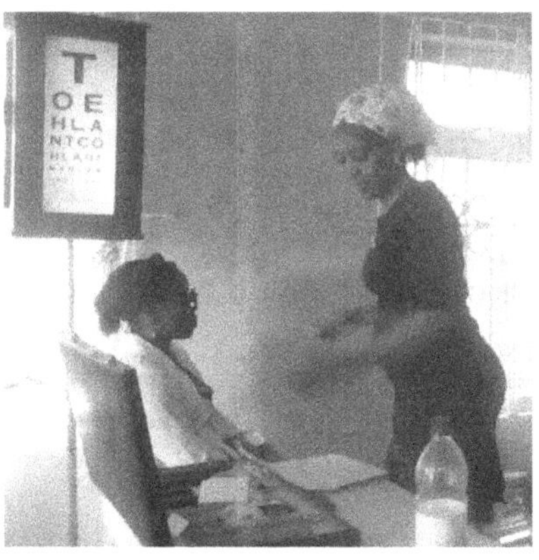

Opticians are technicians, they are professionals in the field of designing, finishing, fitting, and dispensing of eyeglasses and contact lenses, based on an eye doctor prescription, and they also dispense low vision aids and artificial eyes.

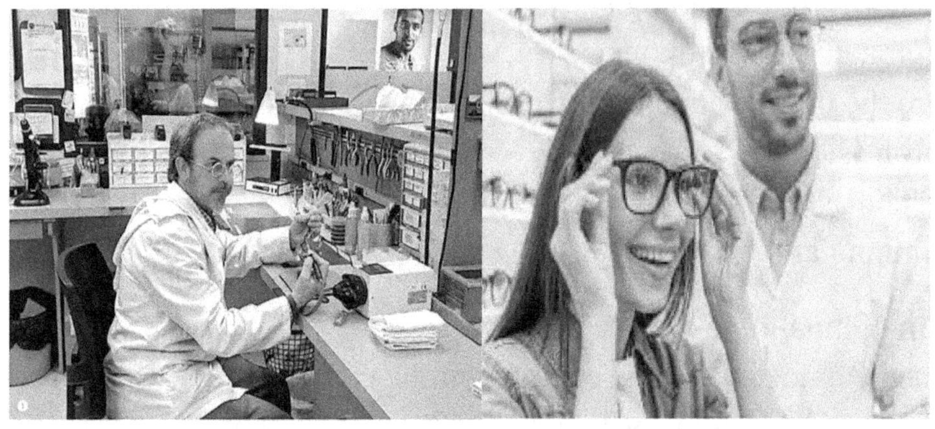

Ophthalmologists and optometrist can further specialize in different fields like pediatric, geriatric, low vision, vision therapy, ocular diseases, etc.

Optometrist and ophthalmologists both perform a routine eye exam and both are trained to detect, diagnose, and manage eye diseases that require medical and non-medical treatment.

Certain eye disorders require care and treatment of an ophthalmologist particularly if surgery or other specialty care is needed. However, an optometrist can also co-manage a surgery patient.

Knowledge about your eye care providers is important, to know the best provider for your needs.

5.3. GENERAL BODY EXAM

It's important to know that the eye is connected to many other systems in the human body, thus routine general body exam is essential for a healthy eye.

General body exams could be performed by a doctor, nurse, or physician assistant.

It helps determine the general status of your health, these exams are used to;

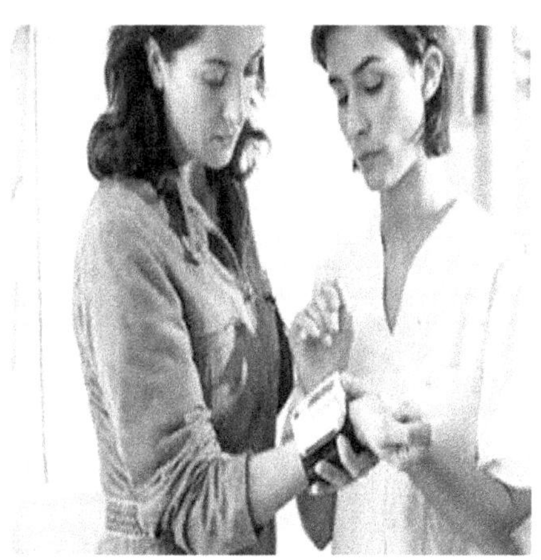

- check blood pressure, pulse rate, temperature, blood sugar, cholesterol level,

- check your weight and height to estimate your body mass index, to avoid obesity,

- check for possible diseases and treat if necessary,

- identify any issue that may become a medical concern in future,

- update necessary immunization,

- ensure that you are maintaining a healthy diet and exercise routine.

Regular screening helps your care provider to treat these conditions before they become severe.

Most health conditions affect our sight and the sooner its detected and treated or managed the better the health of the eyes.

Some of these health conditions that show symptoms in the eyes and endanger it are; hypertension, diabetes, tumors, autoimmune disorders, thyroid disease, sickle cell disease, liver disease, multiple sclerosis, Parkinson's disease, and other neurological or brain disorder.

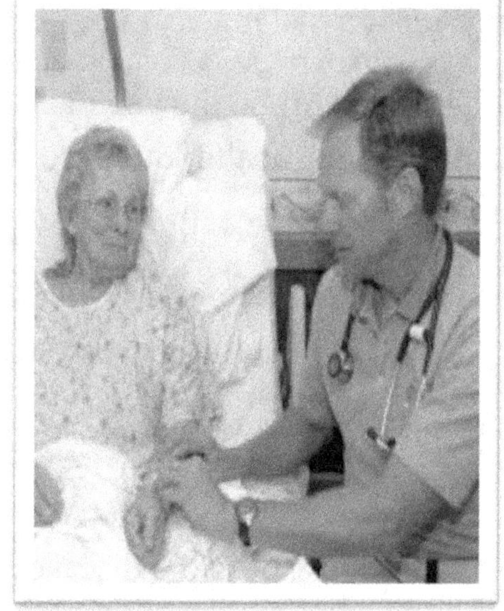

Early detection of these will not only reduce vision loss but also can minimize the risk of complications such as heart diseases, kidney failure, stroke, heart attack, blindness.

It's advisable to have regular checkups because early detection gives you the best chance for getting the right treatment quickly and avoid any complications; it also helps to lower the risk of various health conditions.

Routine health check at least once a year is recommended for a healthier, longer, and happier life.

5.4. FAMILY MEDICAL HISTORY

Being aware of your family medical history is an important part of a lifelong wellness plan.

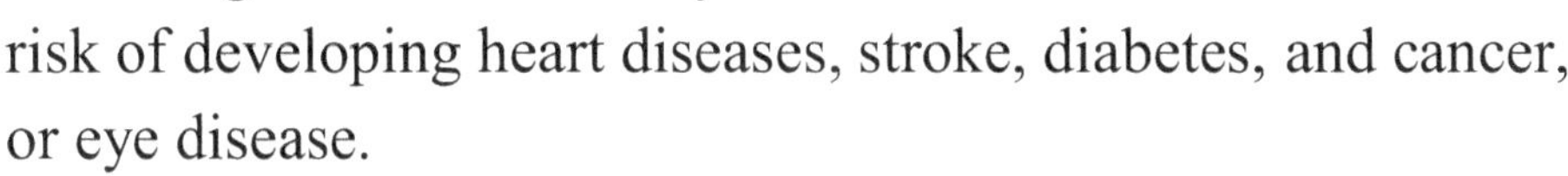

Family medical history is a record of health history about a person and his close relatives.

Family medical history is one of the strongest influences on your risk of developing heart diseases, stroke, diabetes, and cancer, or eye disease.

Even though you cannot change your genetic makeup, knowing your family history can help you reduce your risk of developing health problems.

Family members share their genes as well as their environment, lifestyle, and habits. Everyone can recognize traits such as curly hair, dimples, leanness, or athletic ability that run in their families.

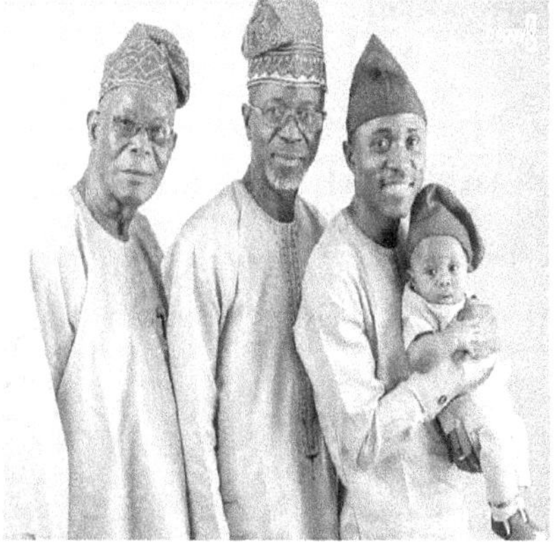

Families have many factors common which can give clues to medical conditions that may run in a family.

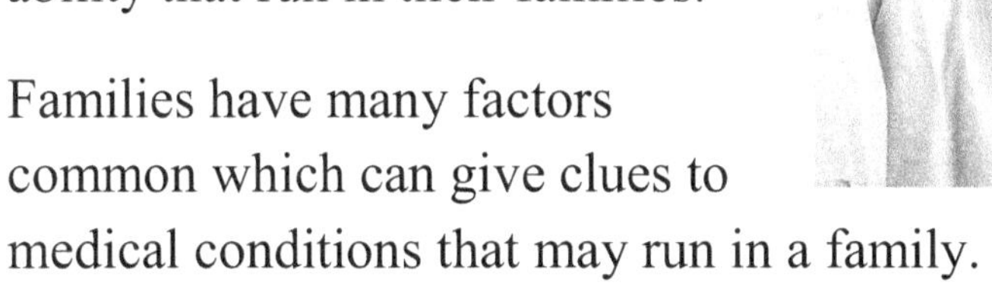

Certain ocular conditions have a strong genetic inheritance example, autosomal dominant retinitis pigmentosa, dominant optic atrophy or an individual may have an increased risk due to a condition affecting a first-degree relative example, primary open-angle glaucoma.

Having a family history of eye diseases can put you at a higher risk for developing one yourself.

Glaucoma diseases can be genetic and can cause blindness, if detected late or left untreated, therefore it's important to know your family history and share it with your doctor.

If you have a family history of eye disease, it's good to schedule an eye exam early, that way you and your doctor can take appropriate preventive steps to minimize your risk and save your sight.

While a family medical history provides information about the risk of specific health concerns, having relatives with a medical condition, does not mean that an individual will develop that condition.

To learn about your family medical history, ask questions, talk at family gatherings, and look at family medical records and death certificates to know the disease cause of death.

Collect information about your grandparents, parents, aunts, uncles, cousins, nieces, nephews, siblings, and children, the complete record includes information from 3 generations.

Share the information with your doctor, who will assess your disease risk based on your family history and other risk factors, recommend lifestyle changes to help prevent diseases, prescribe screening tests to detect diseases early.

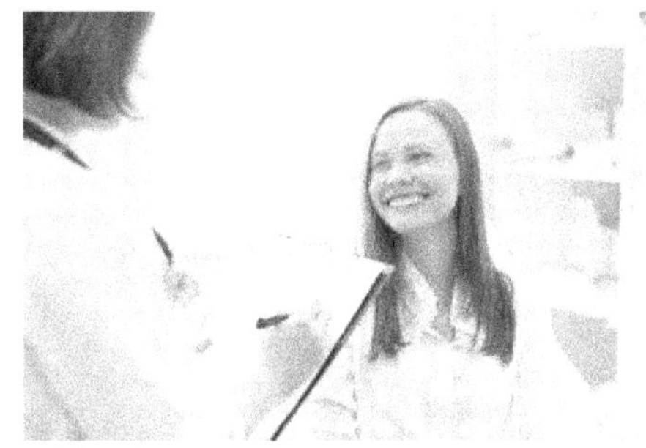

People with a family history of eye diseases may have the most to gain from lifestyle changes and screening tests.

You cannot change your genes but you can change unhealthy behaviors, such as smoking, inactivity, and poor eating habits, this could reduce your risk of diseases that run in your family.

A person with no family history of a disease may still be at risk of developing the disease, therefore adopting a healthy lifestyle is the key to save vision.

5.5. *TOPICAL EYE MEDICATIONS*

Your eyes are sensitive and delicate, visit only your eye care doctors for proper eye examination and use only medication prescribed by them.

Your eye medications could be informed of solutions, suspension, gels, or ointment.

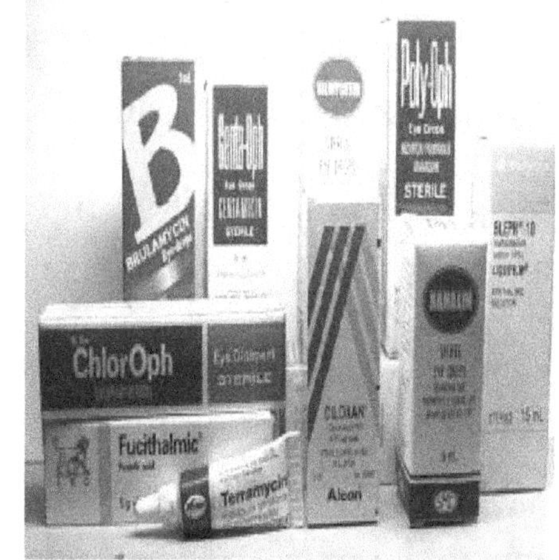

Use your drugs exactly as directed, don't stop just because your eyes feel better, for sometimes stopping a drop too early or abruptly can cause a rebound effect.

Using your medication as prescribed by your eye doctor can increase the success rate of treatment.

Incorrect use of your eye medications can decrease effectiveness, loss of medication (wasting), adverse effects, eye injury (if the tip of the container scratches your eyes), or the medication becomes contaminated.

Always check the expiry date of your medication before buying and do not use or keep it beyond the printed expiry date.

The current policy is once eye medication has been opened, you should discard after 28 days because it might have been contaminated with hands, eyelid, dirt, dust, etc. Note the date you opened it, however, adhere to your doctor's instruction.

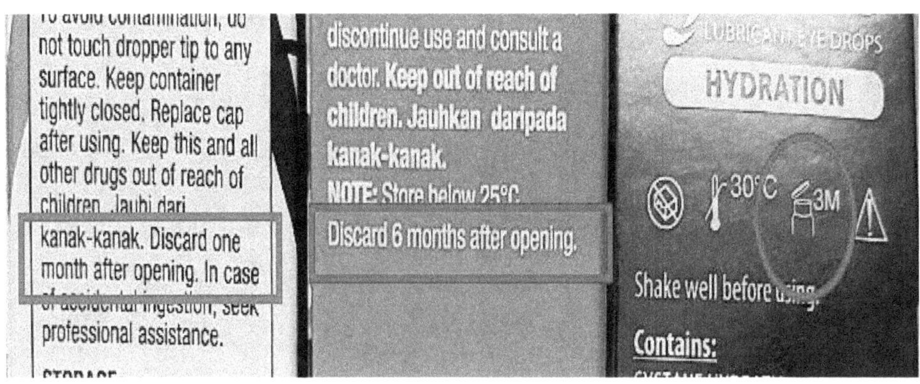

Eye medications need to be stored at a particular temperature, to prevent the ingredients from degrading and becoming less effective.

Always check the medication for recommended storage temperature, generally, they are stored in a cool dry place, but some are preferably stored in the fridge.

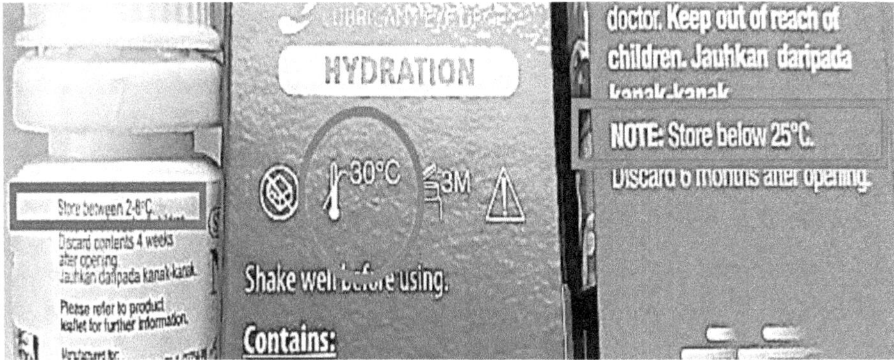

Read the leaflet and instructions on the medication to note the manufacturers and expiry date, storage, side effects, contraindications, and other information.

 Do not instill urine, breastmilk, fuel, or any of such substance into your eyes also avoid self-medication for your eyes it can be dangerous.

Proper topical medication administration;

- Wash your hands thoroughly with soap and clean water and dry with a clean towel.

- You can use the mirror to see what you are doing if you find it helpful.

- Shake the content if recommended, then open and avoid all contact between the tip and your eyes or anything else to avoid its contamination.

- Tilt your head backward, pull down the lower lid of your eye with your index finger to form a pocket, and lookup.

- If the medication is an eye drop, hold the dropper with the other hand and squeeze just one drop into the pocket in the middle of the lower eyelid. Close

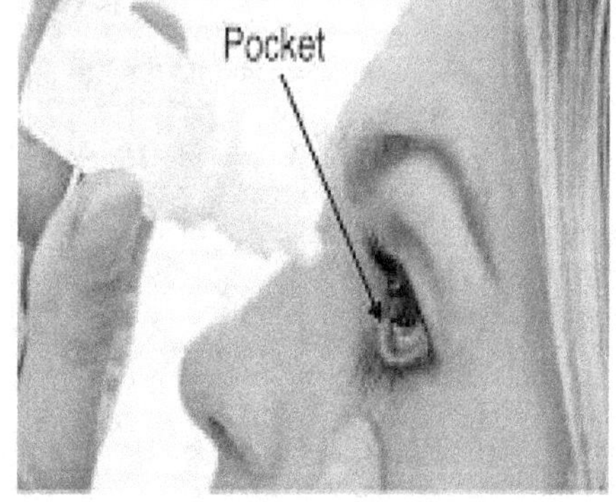

the container after application, to avoid contamination.

- If the medication is an ointment or gel, apply a thin layer all along the inside of the lower eyelid, starting from the inside of the eyelid (from the nose) and continuing towards the outside corner of 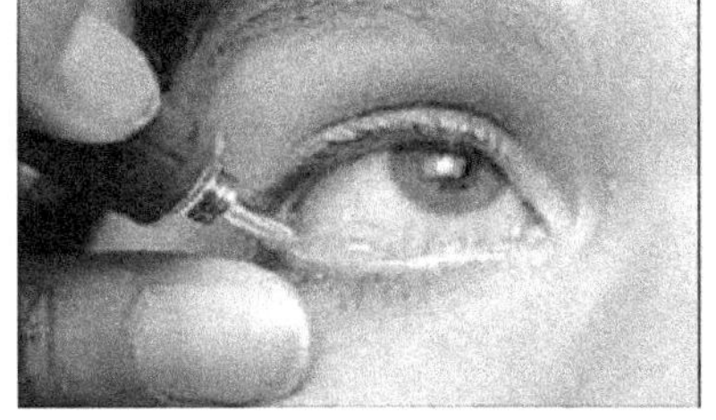 the eyelid. Once the application is done, close the container quickly to avoid content leakage and wastage.

- Bring your head down, close your eyes for about 2-3 minutes to help it absorb properly, try not to blink, or squeeze your eyes.

- Wipe excess product that might have leaked, with a clean tissue, never wipe the tip of your medication to avoid contamination.

- You can place your index finger, along the inner corner of your eye, close to your nose after putting the drops in, this closes off the tear duct and keeps the drops in the eye longer. This increases the effectiveness of the drop and reduces the systemic side effects. 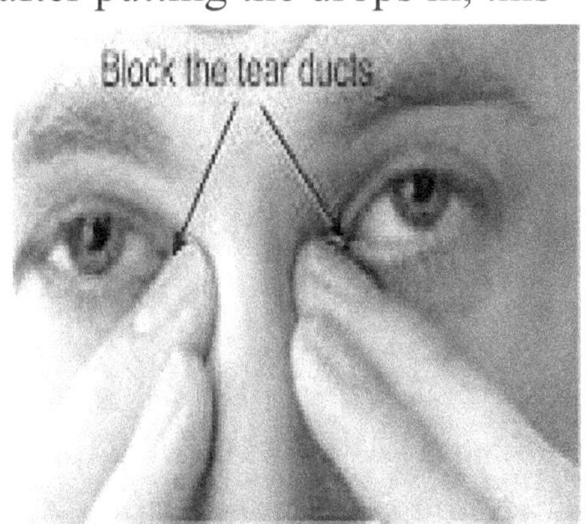

- Wash your hand thoroughly to remove any residue of medication.

Just one drop is enough to fit into your eyelid's eye pocket; the second drop will just run down your cheek.

Wait for 5 – 10mins between each medication. If you are applying multiple medications, otherwise you will wash the first drop out with the second drop, thus reducing its effectiveness.

If you have both eye drops and ointments, use the drops first, if not the ointment may keep the eye drops from being absorbed.

Many eye medications can cause slight stinging sensation after instilling or blurry vision; this is normal and should go away after a few minutes, if not report to your eye doctor immediately.

Remove your contact lens before instilling your eye medication, unless instructed otherwise by your doctor.

Do not share your medication with anyone, to avoid contamination, and also the medication may not be what is needed for the other person.

It's easier to let some else help you administer your medication.

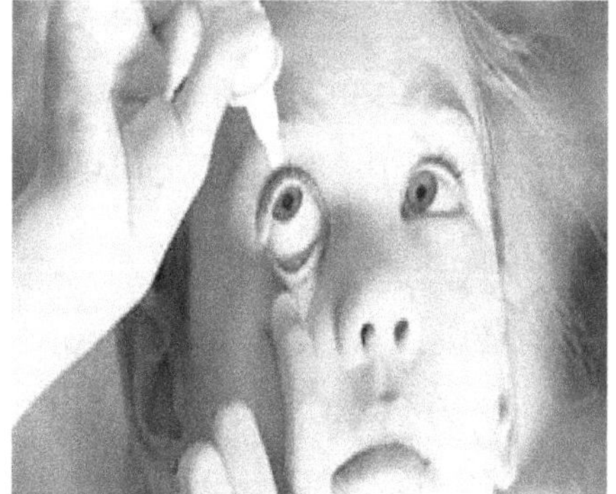

Your eyes are fragile and indispensable; therefore, the correct use of medication is vital to keep them healthy.

CHAPTER 6: OUT DOOR ACTIVITIES

6.1. SUNLIGHT

Sunlight is solar radiation that is visible at earth's surface, it comprises of 3 major components;

- Visible light, wavelength between 0.4-0.8 micrometer

- Ultraviolet light, wavelength shorter than 0.4 micrometers (100-380nm)

- Infrared radiation, wavelength longer than 0.8 micrometers.

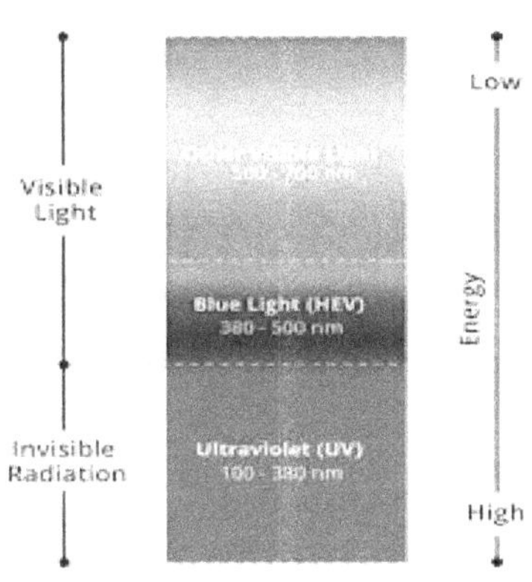

Sunlight contains visible light rays and invisible ultraviolet rays.

Visible light emitted by the sun comprises a range of different colored light rays that contain different amounts of energy.

Blue light is a portion of visible light ranging from 380-500nm it has the shortest wavelength and highest energy.

Sunlight is the main source of blue light, but there are also many man-made, indoor sources such as fluorescent, LED lighting, flat-screen television, display screens of computers, electronic notebook, smartphones, and other digital devices.

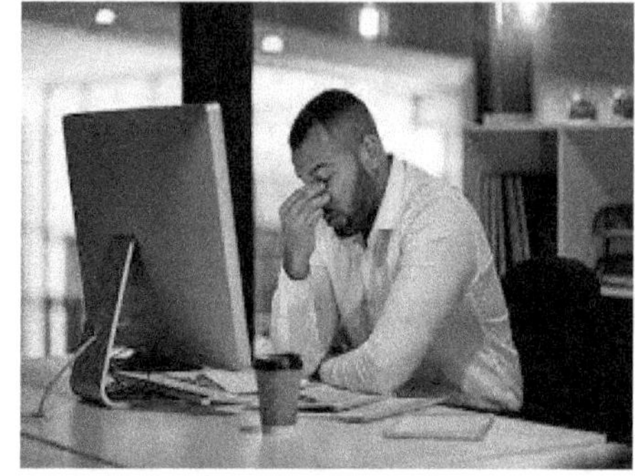

These man-made sources of blue light emit only a fraction of that emitted by the sun, but the amount of time spent using these devices and the proximity of these screens may be harmful to the eyes.

The eye is not very good in blocking blue light, virtually all visible blue light passes through the cornea and the lens and reaches the retina, thus, too much exposure can cause macular degeneration.

Blue light also contributes to digital eye strain, computer glasses, and protective blue light filters on our digital devices are recommended.

However, some blue light exposure is essential for good health, it can boost alertness, help memory and cognitive function, and elevates mood. Blue light regulates circadian rhythm-the the body's natural wakefulness and sleep cycle.

Ultraviolet rays (UV rays) comprises invisible high energy rays from the sun, that lies just beyond the blue end of the visible spectrum.

Although UV light constitutes only a very small proportion of the total radiation, this component is very important.

UV light produces vitamin D, which is involved in maintaining healthy bones, only 15 minutes of sun exposure provides the needed vitamin D.

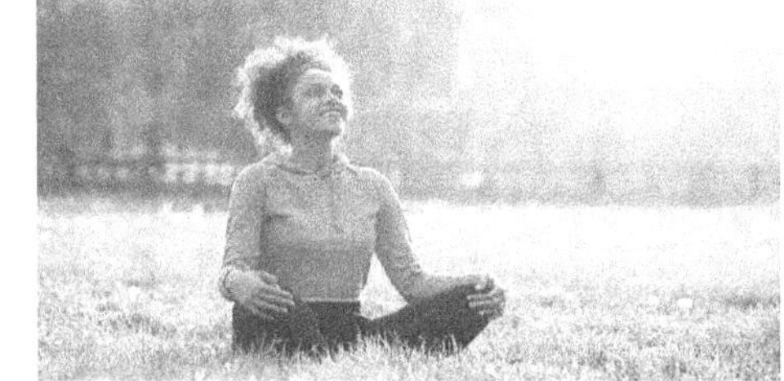

Too much exposure to UV radiation, present in sunlight, is harmful to the eyes and also the skin.

More than 99% of UV rays, is absorbed by the anterior structures of the eye, although some of them do reach the light-sensitive retina.

Damage to the eyes from UV radiation is cumulative, meaning it builds up over our lifetime and can have a permanent effect on our eyes.

UV absorption by the eyes may contribute to the development of age-related cataract and macular degeneration, pterygium, cancer around the eye, photokeratitis, corneal degenerative changes.

Everyone is at risk of developing ocular damage from sun exposure, therefore we need to take special care to protect our eyes and avoid excessive exposure.

Wear a wide-brimmed hat or cap to block the sunray and reduce its absorption to the eyes.

UV absorbing eyewear especially with wraparound design provides the greatest measure of UV protection, wear proper eye protection and hats that block 99-100% of UV rays.

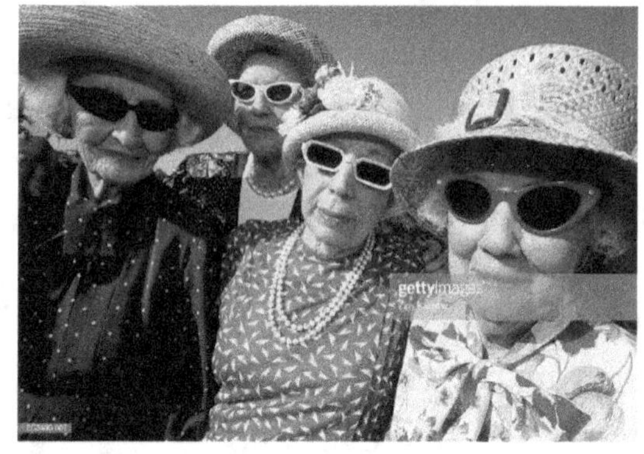

Sun rays can come from many directions, they can reflect from the ground, water, snow, sand, and other bright surfaces, so wear your sunglasses even when you are in a shade.

In cooperate UV protection in your eyewear, both prescription and non-prescription glasses. UV protection includes; UV blocking lens materials, lens coatings, and photochromic.

Even if your contact lens blocks UV rays, you still need sunglasses, because UV rays can still damage your eyelid and other tissues not covered by the lens.

Wear sunglasses that are large enough to shield the eyes from most angles and a hat along with it.

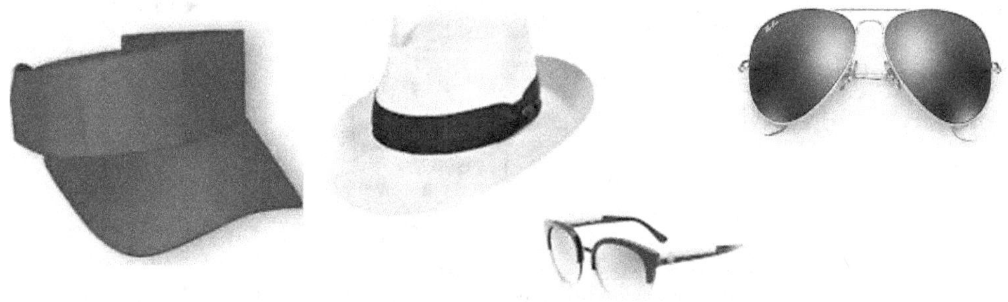

6.2. SEDENTARY LIFESTYLE

A sedentary lifestyle is a type of lifestyle that involves little or no physical activity, which may involve sitting or lying down while carrying out our various activities, for extended periods.

We spend hours sitting during transportation, sitting on our desk at work, sitting or lying down while reading, socializing, watching TV, playing games, using our phones or computers for a long period of hours.

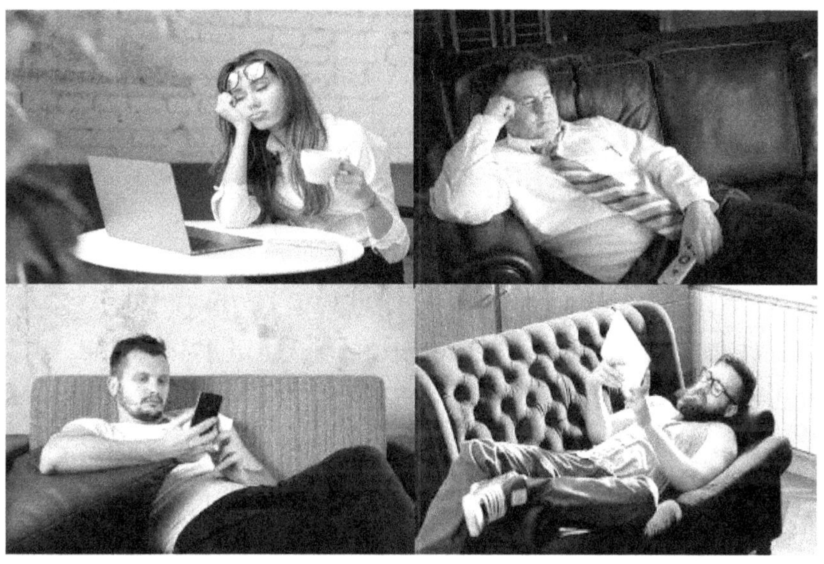

An accumulation of sedentary behaviors for long hours (about 6 hours or more) in a day negatively impacts our health.

Consequences of a sedentary lifestyle include; cardiovascular issues, hypertension, anxiety, depression, diabetes, obesity, lack of sleep, loss productivity, computer eye syndrome, stroke, high cholesterol level.

With advances in technology and transportation, we adopted a more sedentary lifestyle with little or no exercise or activity.

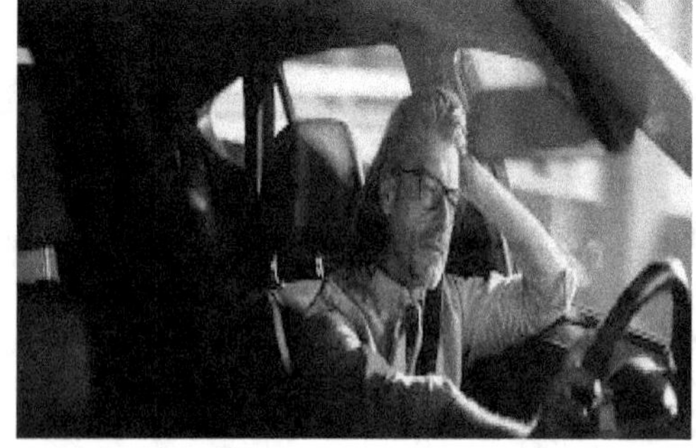

An inactive lifestyle can cause the burning of fewer calories, lose muscle strength, weakness of bones and loss of some mineral content, lower immune system, affect body metabolism, poorer blood circulation, hormonal imbalance, etc.

A sedentary lifestyle can leave a person at greater risk of vision loss as they age than a more active lifestyle, this is because many of those chronic diseases that impact our health can take a toll on our vision.

These eye diseases may include diabetic retinopathy, hypertensive retinopathy, glaucoma, computer vision syndrome, age-related macular degeneration, cataract.

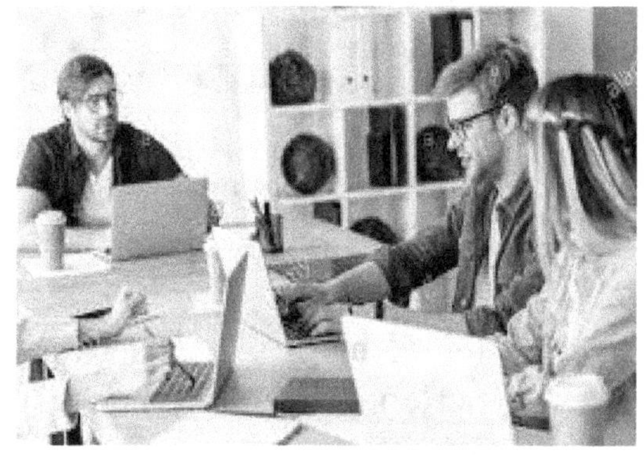

Go for a daily 30 minutes work, try having a walking meeting, instead of sitting at the conference table, always take a stroll daily.

If your job requires you to sit for long periods, stand up at least every 20 minutes, you can set a reminder.

Take the stairs whenever possible instead of the elevator.

Do some home chores like cleaning, washing, sweeping, gardening, and other physical activities, like running, swimming, jogging, and other forms of exercise.

Make it a point of duty to take small breaks from your work to move around, it will help reduce the amount of time you spend sedentary each day.

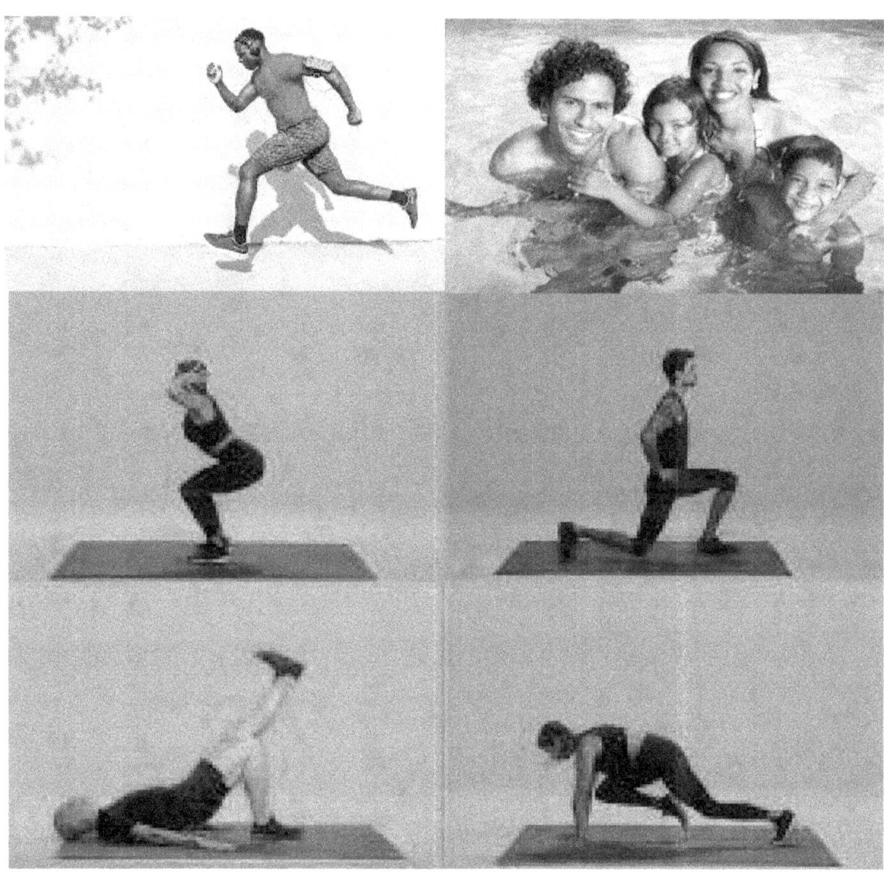

6.3. EXERCISE

Staying active is crucial to overall health, exercise can help you focus, lose weight, tone your muscles, improve energy levels, lower blood pressure, it can also protect your eyesight.

Hormones and anti-oxidants that are known to combat the effects of cell damage in the body, including the eyes are released to the body by exercising.

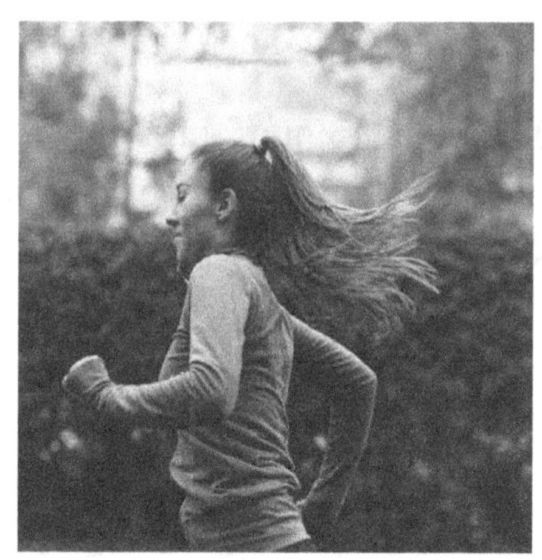

Exercise improves blood circulation, which improves oxygen levels to the eyes and removal of toxins.

Regular exercise can help reduce the risk of some eye diseases and protect your eyes as you age.

Getting regular exercise may not directly affect your eyesight; it may affect other health issues like diabetes, high blood pressure, high cholesterol levels, which are linked to many eye diseases, which could cause vision loss.

Regular exercise can help reduce eye pressure and increase blood flow to the optic nerve and retina.

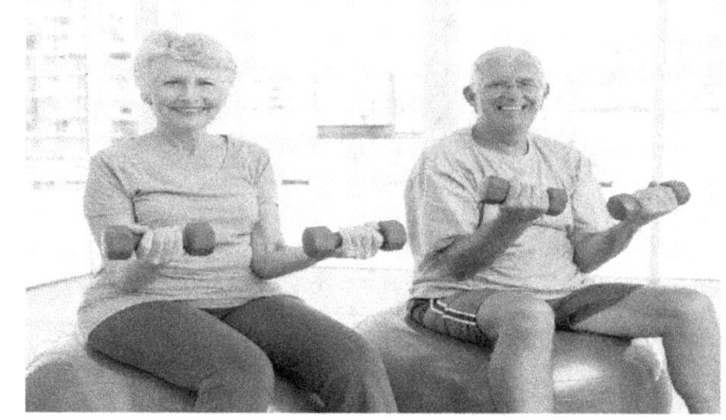

This is more beneficial to people with glaucoma.it can also reduce the risk of eye diseases, like cataract, glaucoma, and wet age-related macular degeneration.

Schedule for regular exercise 3 or more times per week, maybe for about 30 minutes.

Exercise could be taking a brisk walk, jogging, bike riding, dancing, climbing the stairs, running, swimming, thus moderation is the key.

Regular exercise keeps you and your eyes healthy and helps to avoid serious health conditions, so make exercise a priority.

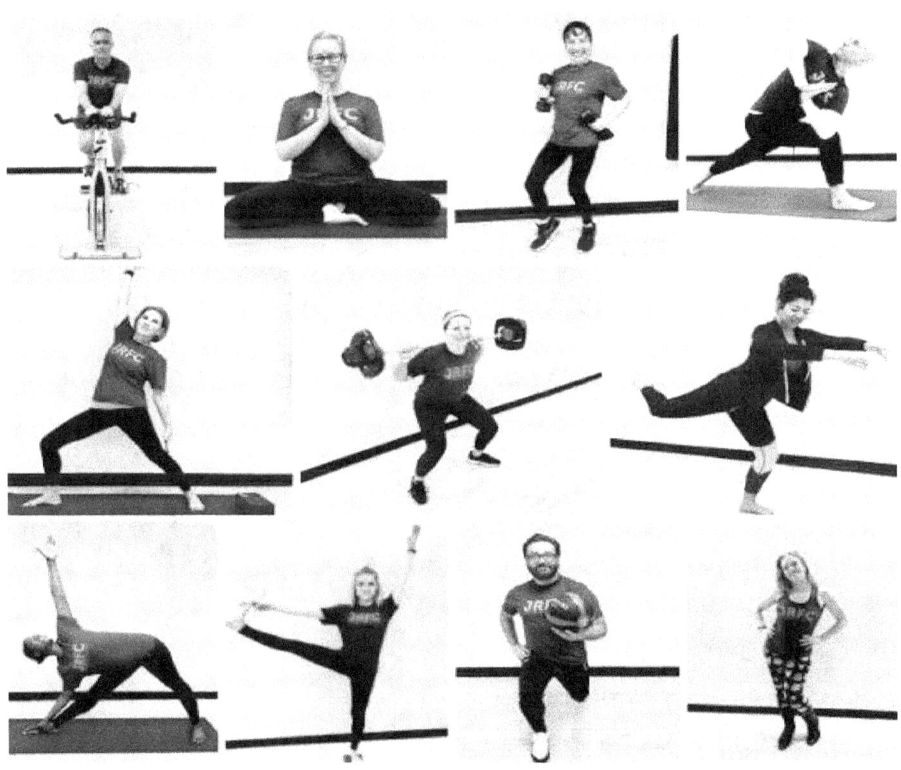

7.1. DIGITAL DEVICES

With the invention of technology, a lot of people use digital devices like computers, tablets, smartphones, for longer periods in the offices or working from home.

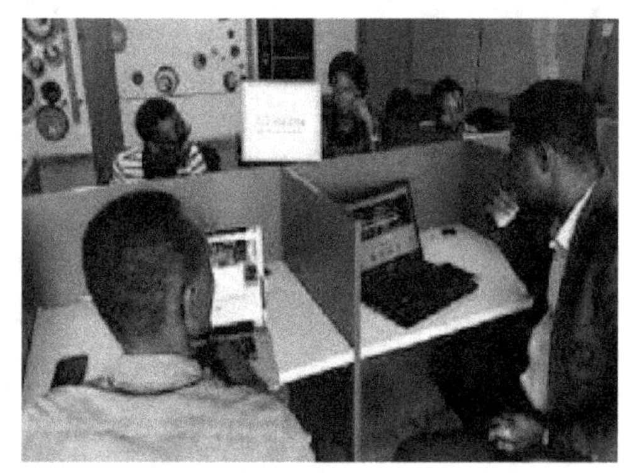

We live in a digital world; extended screen time is quickly becoming a norm in our everyday lives.

The digital screen gives off little or no harmful radiation, thus its level of discomfort or harm appears to increase with the amount of time spent on the screen and proximity of the screen.

The digital screen does expose your eyes to blue light. Blue light exposure you get from the screen is small compared to that gotten from the sun.

Viewing digital screens pushes the eyes to work harder, leading to high visual demands, this is because letters on the screens are not as sharply or precisely defined as those on printed pages, reducing the contrast between them and the background.

Many individuals experience eye discomfort and vision problems, including neck, back and shoulder ache, when viewing digital screens for an extended period, however, it's advisable to avoid long hours with digital screens.

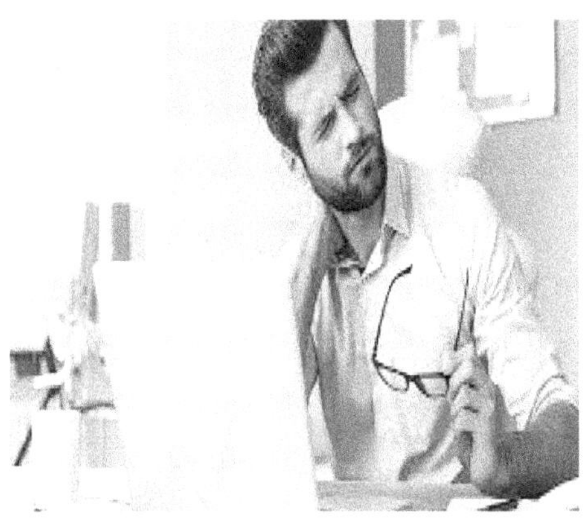

The most common symptoms associated with computer vision syndromes are eyestrain, headaches, blurred vision, dry eyes, shoulder, and neck pain, which may be caused by;

- Poor lighting

- Glare on a digital screen

- Improper viewing distances

- Poor seating posture

- Uncorrected vision problems

- A combination of these factors.

Some important factors in preventing or reducing the symptoms of computer vision syndrome have to do with how it's used;

- Always take breaks when using your devices, follow the 20-20-20 rule;

- Take a 20second break every 20mins and look at something 20 feet away.it helps to relax the eye muscles responsible for focusing at near, thereby reducing overall eye fatigue. You can set an alarm as a reminder.

- Place the computer screen 12-20 degrees below eye level (4-5 inches) as measured from the center of the screen and 20-28 inches from the eyes.

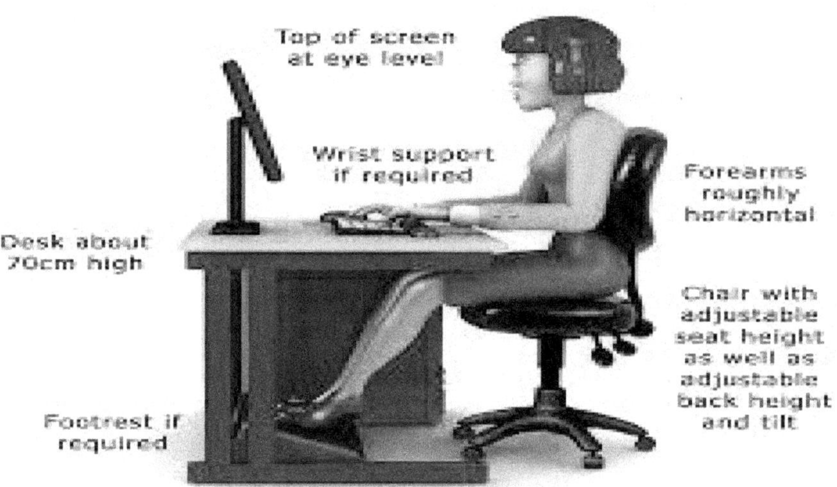

- Have the reference material located below the monitor but above the keyboard or use a document holder beside the monitor to keep you from moving your head when going from document to screen and back.

- To avoid glare, position your screen away from overhead lighting or window.

- Adjust screen brightness to have it approximately the same as your surrounding area and adjust text contrast and size for comfort.

- Sit on a padded chair that conforms to your body at heights where your feet are resting flat on the floor.

It's important to have a comprehensive eye exam at least once a year, to prevent or treat computer vision problems.

If you use prescribed glasses it's good to wear glasses with anti-reflective coating, it helps reduce glare. Reduce your exposure with regular breaks and consider computer glasses to help reduce your exposure to potentially harmful blue light emitted by digital devices.

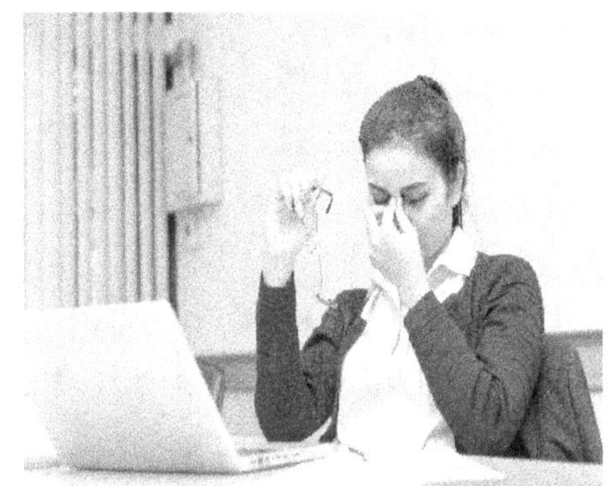

7.2. BLINKING

Blinking is a bodily function, it's a rapidly closing and opening of the eyelid.it could be voluntary or involuntary.

It's an essential function of the eyes, it provides moisture to the eyes by irrigation, using tears, and a lubricant the eye secretes, it regulates and spread tears 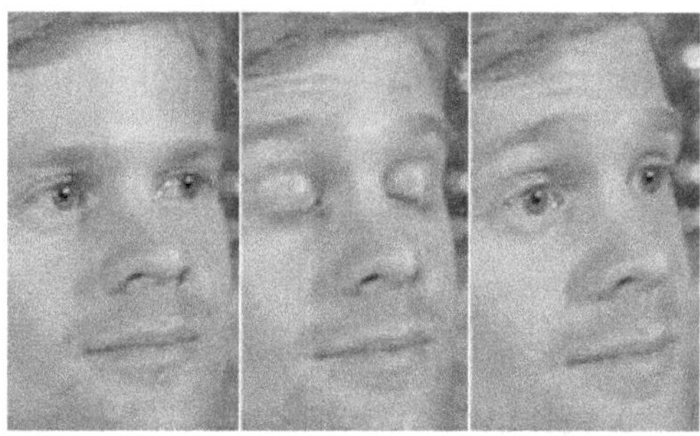 which nourish your eyes with oxygen and nutrients, keeping your eyes healthy and comfortable.

Blinking it's a normal reflex that protects the eyes from dryness, bright light, and foreign body coming towards it. It also cleanses the surface of the eye of any debris and washes it out with fresh tears.

Newborns blink two times per minute and this increases to 14-17 times per minute in adolescence till the remainder of life. Blinking, it's also thought to serve as a momentary rest for the brain.

The coating of tears, by blinking, helps sharpen your vision, clearing and brightening the image your retina receives.

Blinking is also important for contact lens wearers, it helps keep your eyes from itching or irritated, can cut down on the amount of solution or eye drops you need to use and can provide cleaner contact lens accompanied by better vision.

Sometimes being too engrossed in your work especially with digital devices, you tend to forget to blink and rest the eyes; your blink rate typically decreases, meaning you are losing out on cleaning and nourishment of the eyes.

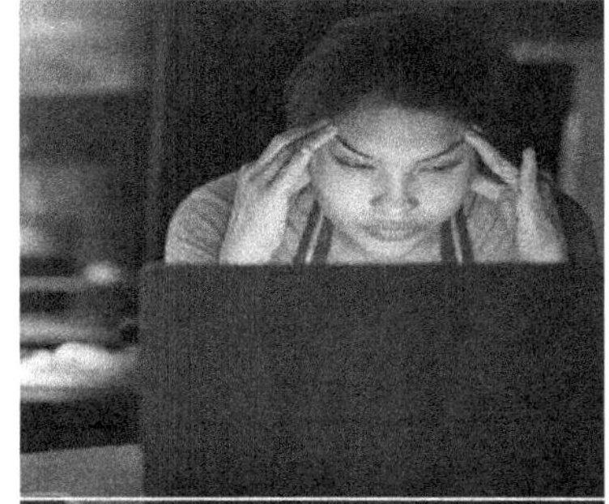

Making a conscious effort to blink every 10-15 seconds will keep your vision sharper while you work and prevent your eyes from feeling strained at the end of your work.

Tears coating the eye evaporate more rapidly during long non-blinking phases and this can place you at a higher risk of dry eyes, eye infection, and eye discomfort and would decrease clarity.

Also, the air in many office environments is dry, which can increase how quickly your tears evaporate, placing you at a greater risk for dry eye problems.

Practice blinking exercise daily;

- Set aside 5 one-minute sessions, spread throughout the day, every day for weeks to blink.

- During each minute, look at 5 different directions (up, down, left, right, center) and blink 10 times in each direction.

- While blinking, make sure your eyes are closing fully, but don't squeeze your lids tight.

7.3. SAFETY EYE WEARS

Eye injuries in the workplace are very common; the right eye protection can lessen the severity or even prevent 90% of these eye injuries.

Workers experience eye injuries if they are not wearing eye protection or wearing the wrong kind of protection for the job.

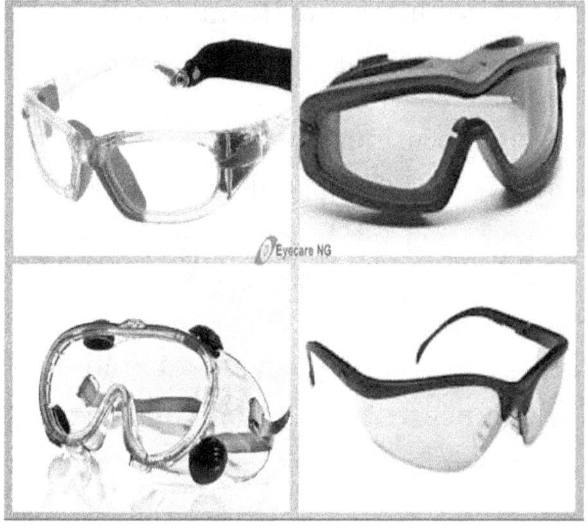

Wear safety eyewear's whenever you are working or passing through areas that pose danger to your eyes. The type of safety eyewear to wear depends on the type of hazard you are exposed to in your workplace.

Safety eye wears are protective eye wears or devices worn to keep the eyes safe from hazards which can cause injuries to the eyes.

Safety eye wears protection includes non-prescription safety glasses, goggles, face shields, welding helmets, full face respiration.

Eliminate hazards before starting work by using machine guards, work screens, or other equipment controls to make the work environment as safe as possible.

Occupations with a high risk of eye injuries include; construction, manufacturing, mining, carpentry, automatic repair, electrical work, plumbing, welding, maintenance.

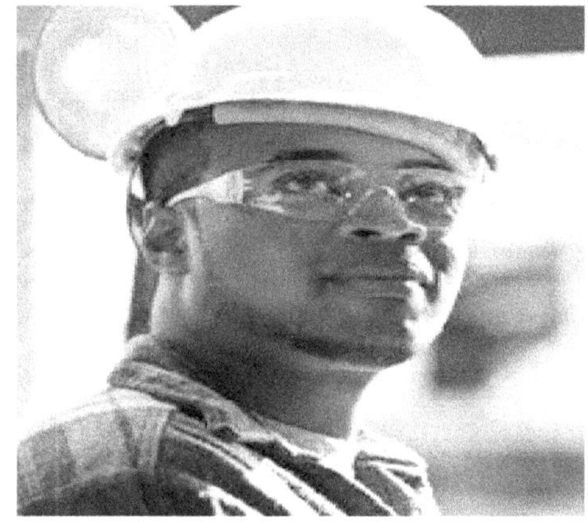

Know the eye hazards at your workplace to help you avoid injuries and use the right safety eyewear designed for the specific duty or hazard.

Common hazards that may cause eye injuries are;

- Projectiles (dust, glasses, concrete, metal, wood and other particles),

- Chemicals (splashes and fumes)

- Harmful radiation (visible light, UV radiation, heat or infrared radiation and lasers)

- Bloodborne pathogens (hepatitis, HIV) from blood and body fluids,

- Tools

Scratched and dirty safety eye wears reduce vision, cause glare, and may contribute to accidents, thus keep them in good condition and replace if damaged and they must fit properly to provide adequate protection.

Visit your eye doctor for an eye exam to avoid accidents which may be caused by uncorrected vision problems or diseases.

Eye protection is mandatory in all areas with the potential for eye injury. Wear the appropriate type of protective eyewear if it's required as part of your job at all times and encourage your co-workers to do so.

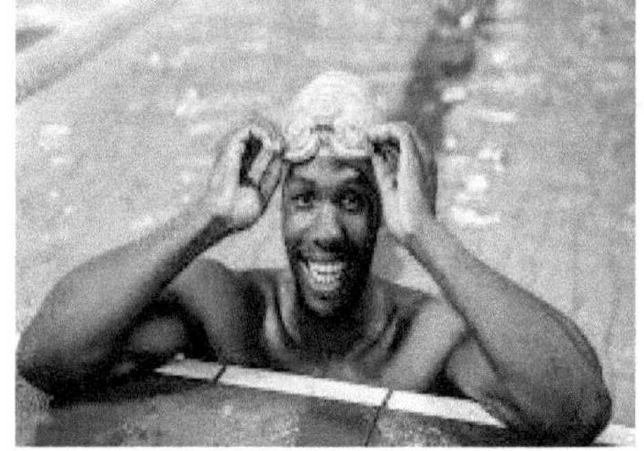

Wear eye protection to prevent injuries during sports, swimming, or doing activities at homes such as home repair, gardening, and cleaning.

Selection of protective eyewear appropriate for a given task should be based on the hazard assessment of each activity;

- Wear wraparound safety glasses or safety glasses with side shields for protection against particles, flying objects, or dust, wear goggles in a severe dusty environment.

- For protection against heat hazards (such as splashes of boiling water, hot oil, steam, open flames or heated ovens or furnace) wear heat resistant safety eye wears, high-temperature face shields worn over a safety glasses or goggles will protect the eyes and other parts of the face.

- Radiation hazards emit intense light and glare, which can enter the eyes and cause retinal burns, cataract and macular degeneration, protection of the eyes requires devices (like, special-purpose glasses, goggles, face shields or helmets) designed for the task and adequately filters the harmful light in each case depending on the type and intensity.

- For chemicals, wear safety goggles that form a complete seal around the eyes. It may also be necessary to prevent inhalation by putting on respiratory safety devices.

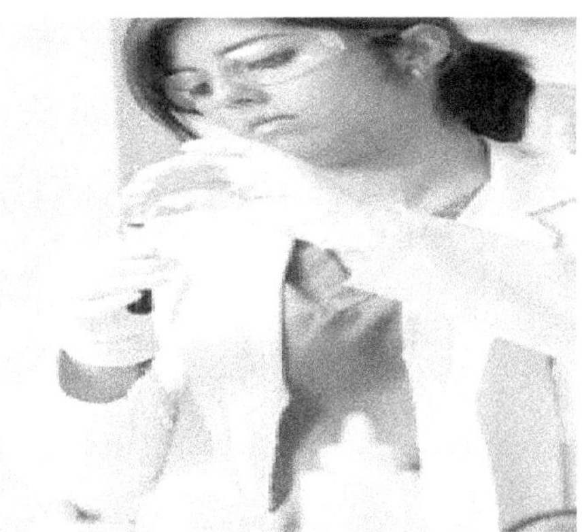

First aid procedures for eye injuries;
- Chemicals;
  - Flush the eyes immediately with water for at least 15 minutes and if you are wearing contact lenses remove them before flushing the eyes.
  - Do not bandage the eyes.
  - Seek immediate medical attention from an eye doctor, after flushing the eyes.
- Particles;
  - Do not rub the eyes, rather blink gently to let your tears wash the speck out or irrigate the eye with artificial tear solution.
  - If the particle did not come out, visit your eye doctor immediately.
- Blows;
  - To reduce pain and swelling, gently apply cold compress or ice on the closed eyelid without applying pressure on the eye, then visit your eye doctor.
  - For cuts and punctures to the eye or eyelid, seek immediate medical attention from your eye doctor.

CHAPTER 8: SOME COMMON EYE PROBLEMS

Farsightedness (hyperopia)

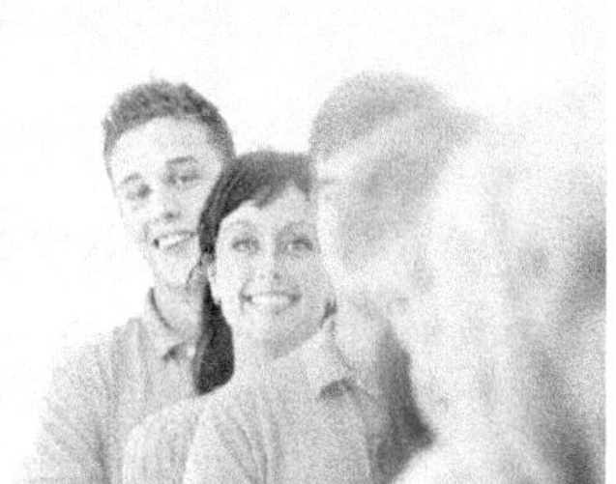

Nearsightedness(myopia)

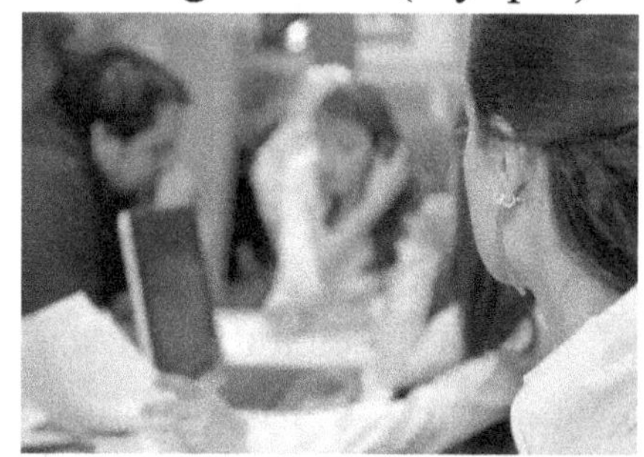

Astigmatism

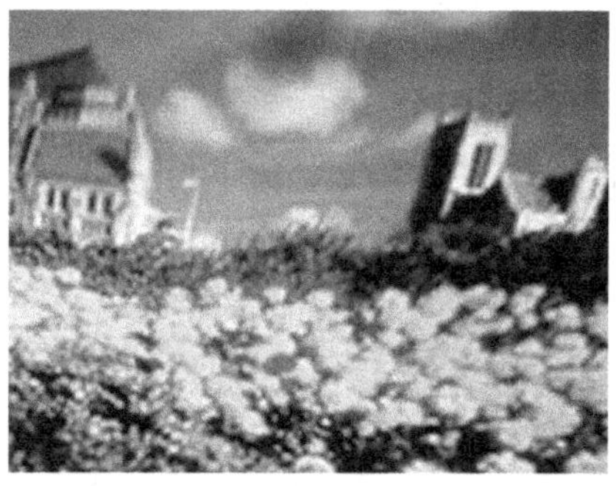

Strabismus

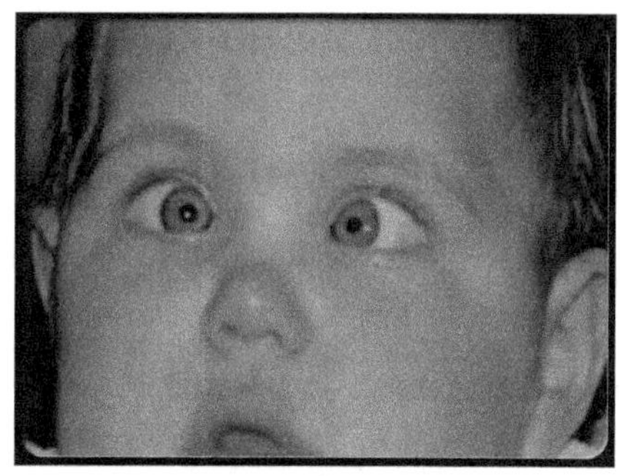

Stye

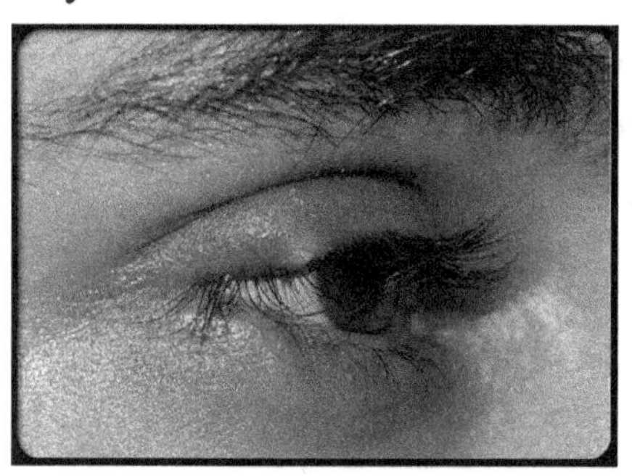

Chalazion

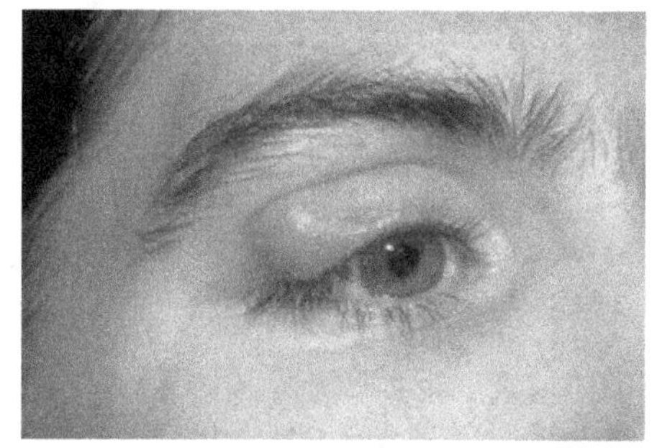

Glaucoma

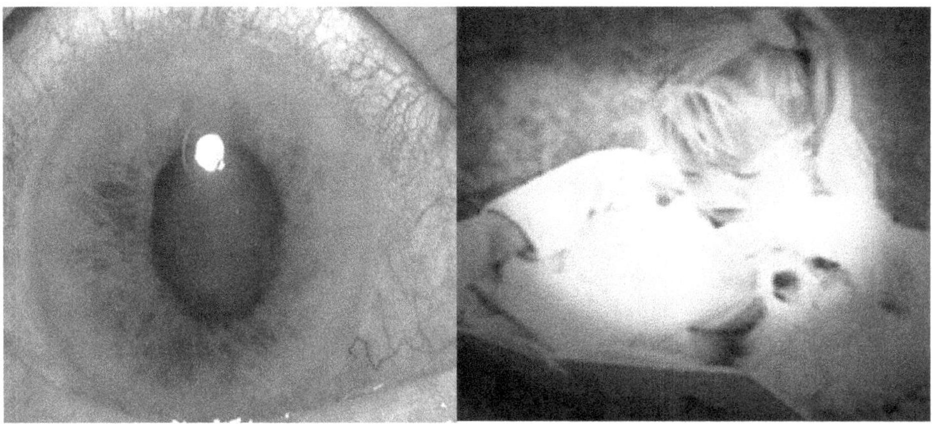

Cataract

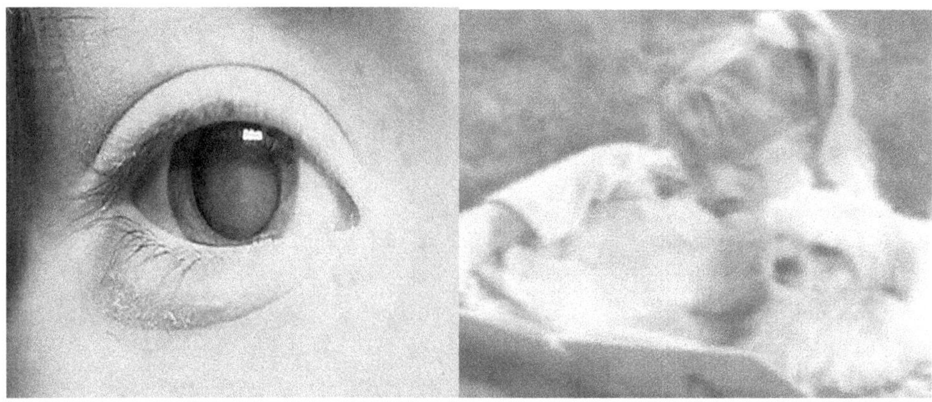

Age-related macular degeneration

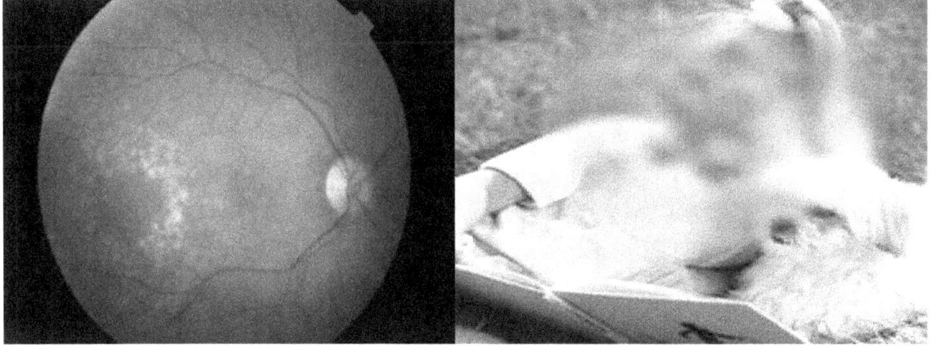

Diabetic retinopathy

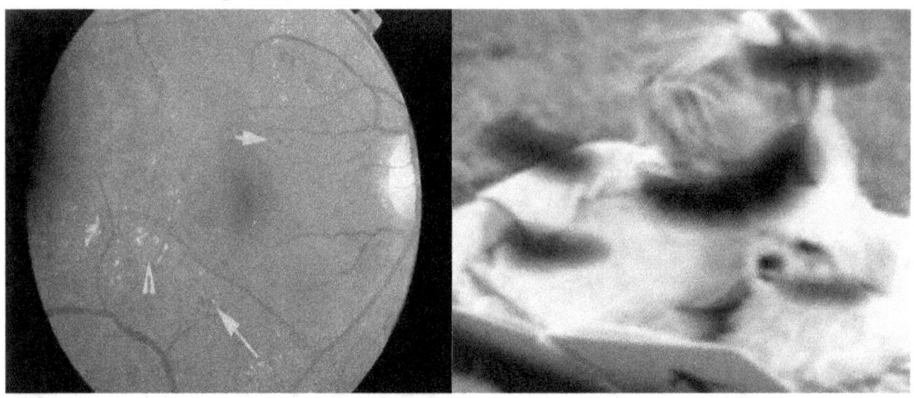

Retinal detachment

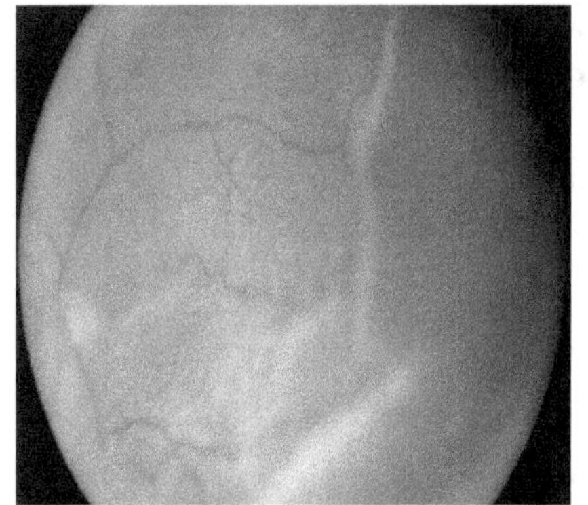

Uveitis

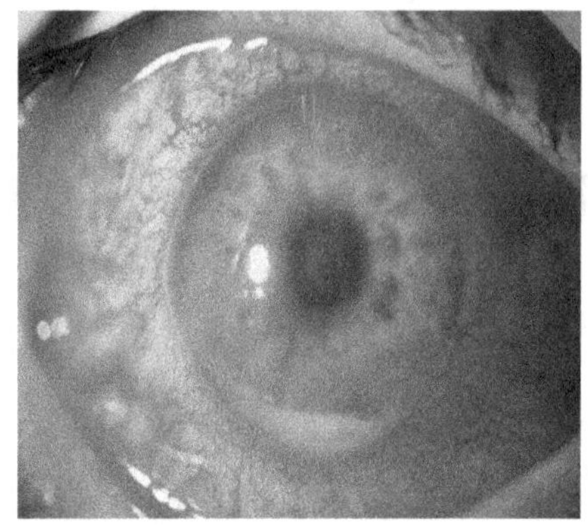

Bacterial conjunctivitis

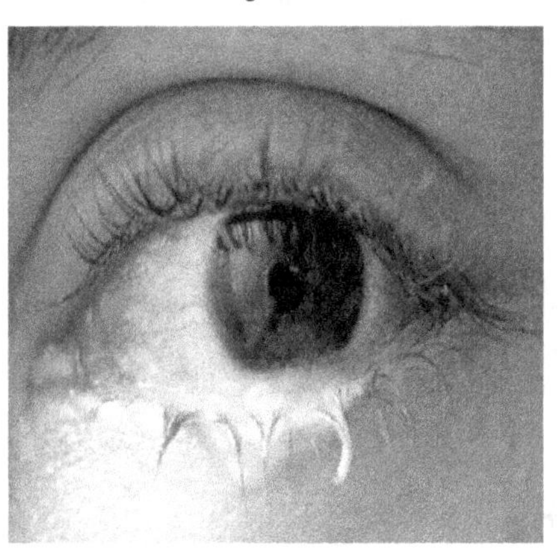

Allergic conjunctivitis

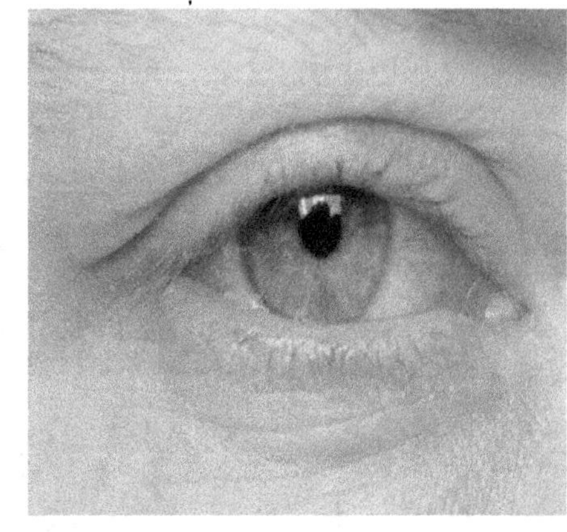

Keratoconus

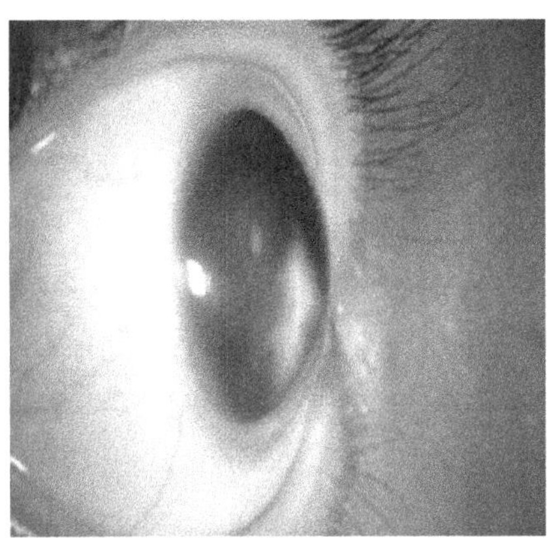

Corneal ulcer

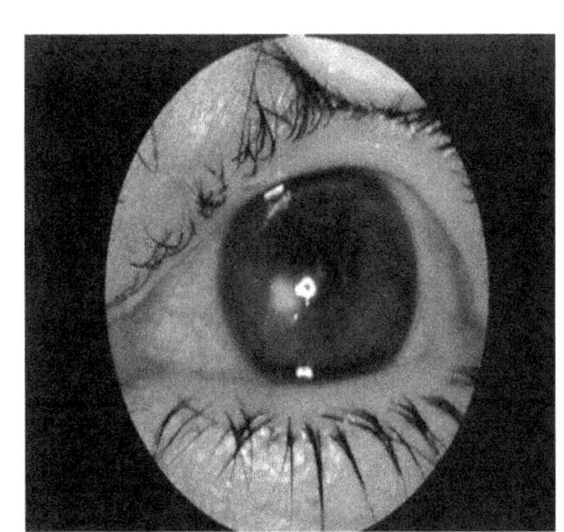

Blepharitis

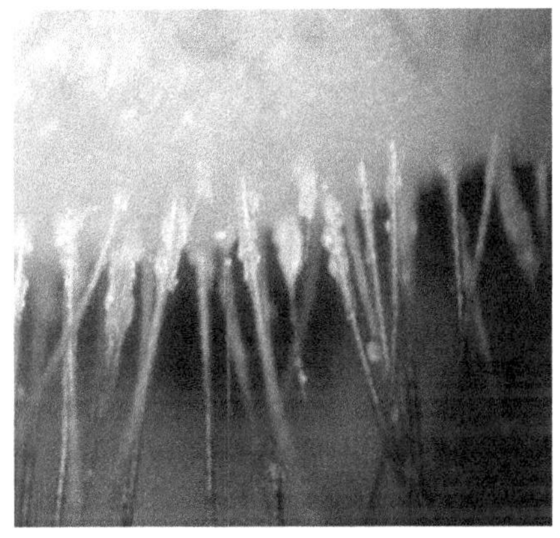

Floaters

Pinguecula

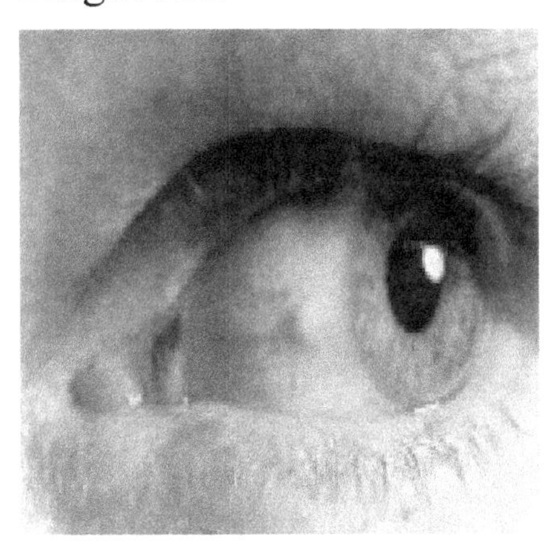

Pterygium

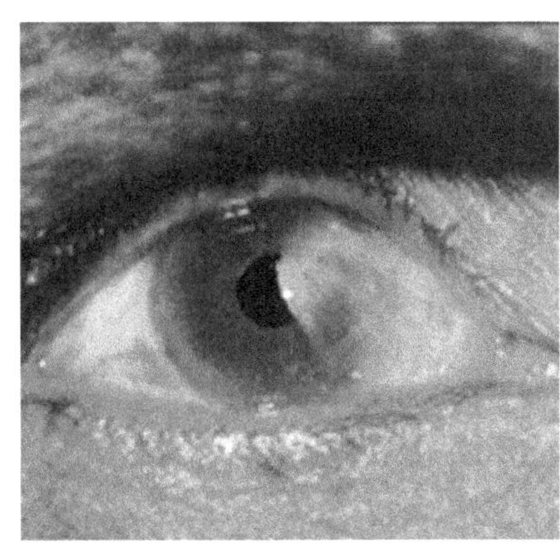

ABOUT THE AUTHOR

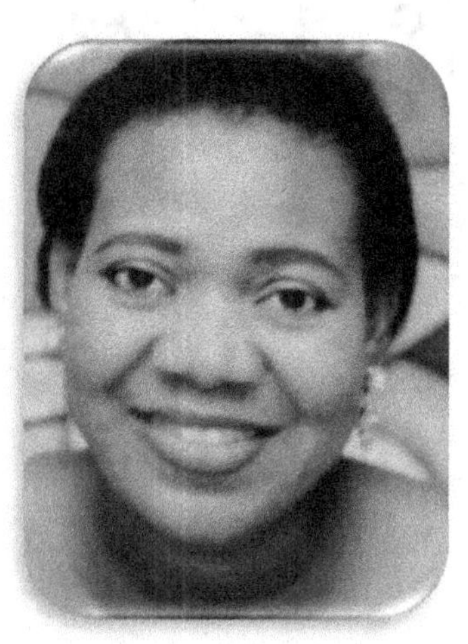

Dr (Mrs.) Menma Angelina Okechukwu is an optometrist and a member of the Nigerian Optometric Association. She is currently the medical director of EMMANUEL CATHOLIC EYE CLINIC.

She graduated from Imo state university in 2012, where she studied optometry, which earned her the certificate of Doctor of Optometry. Her being an eye doctor is a calling by God, who led her to this profession.

Dr. Menma has been working in this profession since 2012, rendering comprehensive and quality eye care services, creating awareness about eye care through educational lectures and giving hope to the hopeless, in her passionate desire to beat blindness, with a slogan **"never give up on any eye"**.

She is a Nigerian and happily married to Engr.Stanley Okechukwu Udeobi and together with their kids, lives, and works in Nigeria.

Dr. Menma is a diligent, hardworking, and humble lady, who never gives up on her goal. However, her passion moved her to write this book to reach out to the masses, for their optimal health.

9 798663 343633